Mental Health and Gr Factsheets

Fourth Edition

Mental Health and Growing Up Factsheets

Fourth Edition

Edited by the Royal College of Psychiatrists'
Child and Family Public Education
Editorial Board

Series Editor: Dr Vasu Balaguru

RCPsych Publications

RCPsych Publications is an imprint of the Royal College of Psychiatrists,
17 Belgrave Square, London SW1X 8PG
www.rcpsych.ac.uk

British Library Cataloguing-in-Publication Data.
A catalogue record for this book is available from the British Library.
ISBN 978 1 908020 46 8

Distributed in North America by Publishers Storage and Shipping Company.

Printed by Bell & Bain Limited, Glasgow, UK.

These factsheets may be photocopied and the photocopies distributed free of charge as long as no profit is gained from their use. Permission to reproduce the factsheets in any other way must be obtained from permissions@rcpsych.ac.uk.

For a catalogue of public education materials or copies of our leaflets contact: Book Sales/Leaflets, The Royal College of Psychiatrists, 17 Belgrave Square, London SW1X 8PG. Email: leaflets@rcpsych.ac.uk, tel: 020 7235 2351 ext. 6146.

These factsheets reflect the best possible evidence at the time of writing.

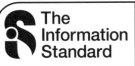

	This organisation has been certified as a producer of reliable health and social care information. www.theinformationstandard.org

The Royal College of Psychiatrists was certified in 2009 as a producer of reliable health and social care information.

Contents

Contributors

1 Bipolar disorder
Information for young people

This is one in a series of factsheets for young people, with practical, up-to-date information about mental health problems (emotional, behavioural and psychiatric disorders) that can affect children and young people.

This factsheet gives some basic information about bipolar disorder and advice on how to get help.

What are the symptoms?

In bipolar disorder you can have:

- manic or hypomanic periods (or 'episodes') also known as 'highs'
- depressive periods (or episodes) also known as 'lows'
- mixed periods (or episodes) when symptoms of both 'highs' and 'lows' happen at the same time.

There are different types of bipolar disorder depending on how severe the symptoms are or how long they last.

The mood changes can sometimes happen very rapidly within hours or days ('rapid cycling'). For some people, the mood symptoms are less severe ('cyclothymia'). In between the highs and lows, there are usually 'normal' periods that can last for weeks or months. However, for some people, especially when they have had the disorder from some time, these periods of 'normalcy' can be shorter or difficult to see.

Below is a list of the sort of symptoms that can occur in each type of episode. You need to have at least one manic or hypomanic episode to be diagnosed with bipolar disorder. You need to have several symptoms at the same time for at least several days. If you have only one symptom, then it is unlikely to be bipolar disorder.

Symptoms that can occur during a 'high' or manic episode

- Feeling incredibly happy or 'high' in mood, or very excited
- Feeling irritable
- Talking too much – increased talkativeness
- Racing thoughts
- Increased activity and restlessness
- Difficulty concentrating, constant changes in plans
- Overconfidence and inflated ideas about yourself or your abilities
- Feeling you need less sleep
- Not looking after yourself
- Increased sociability or overfamiliarity
- More sexual energy than usual
- Overspending of money, or other types of reckless or extreme behaviour.

Hypomania is a milder form of mania (less severe and for shorter periods). During these periods you can feel very productive and creative and so see these experiences as positive and valuable. However, hypomania, if left untreated, can become more severe, and may be followed by an episode of depression. At the extreme end, some people also develop psychosis.

What is bipolar disorder?

Bipolar disorder is also sometimes called manic depression, bipolar affective disorder or bipolar mood disorder, or simply bipolar. It is an illness in which there are extreme changes or swings in mood.

Everyone has times in their life when they feel very happy (such as when you are about to go on holiday) or very sad (such as when your pet dies). But it only becomes a disorder when the mood changes are unusual or extreme. This can range from being unusually happy (known as 'mania' or 'hypomania'), to being unusually sad ('depression') for no apparent cause.

What causes it?

Although the causes are not fully understood, bipolar disorder tends to run in families. In people who have bipolar disorder, episodes may happen at times of stress or disrupted sleep.

How common is it?

Bipolar disorder is extremely rare in young children, but there are quite a few studies that suggest that it may start in teenage years and in early adult life. It affects about 1 in 100 adults.

Symptoms that can occur during a 'low' or depressive episode

- Feeling very sad most of the time
- Less energy and less active
- Not being able to enjoy things you normally like doing
- Lack of appetite
- Disturbed sleep
- Thoughts of self-harm or suicide.

On the milder end, you may just feel sad and gloomy all the time. Here too, at the extreme end, some people can develop psychosis.

Symptoms that can occur during a mixed episode

- A mixture of manic symptoms and depressive symptoms at the same time.

What effects can bipolar disorder have?

The exaggerated thoughts, feelings and behaviours can affect many aspects of your life and can lead to, for example:

- loss of confidence
- loss of a sense of control you have over your life
- poor concentration which affects your academic performance
- problems with relationships with family and friends
- behaviour that could place your health or life at risk, such as drinking alcohol or misusing drugs.

> **Christina, 16**
>
> 'I was a happy, confident person studying for 11 GCSEs and enjoying a good social life with a large circle of friends. All seemed well in my life. Suddenly, from feeling really cheerful, happy and full of energy, I withdrew to my room, stopped eating and stopped talking to everybody, even my parents. I was having vivid hallucinations, became paranoid and even thought about hurting myself.
>
> My parents became really worried and eventually I was admitted to a child and adolescent psychiatric unit. I now realise that I had mania before I plunged into black depression. Once I was diagnosed with bipolar disorder, I was able to understand and come to terms with my illness. Medication was given to me to deal with the mood swings, together with a talking therapy.
>
> With support from my family and friends, I am now back at school and I hope to go to medical school in the next couple of years.' ✪

How is it treated?

In the short term, depending on whether you are high or low and how severe it is, you may need different treatments. When you have severe symptoms, you may need medications and also sometimes admission to hospital to help your symptoms, and also keep you safe. In the long term, the goal of treatment is to help you have a healthy, balanced and productive life. This would include understanding the condition, controlling the symptoms and stopping the illness from coming back.

- **Help with understanding yourself and the illness (psychoeducation)**

  It is very important that you and your family are helped to understand bipolar disorder, how best to cope and what to do to reduce the chances of it coming back. You and your family may notice 'triggers' to your episodes and/or early warning signs that an episode is starting. Being aware of these can help reduce the chance of episodes occurring, and getting help in the earliest stages of an episode can stop it from getting worse.

- **Talking treatments (also known as psychological therapies)**

  These may include different types of therapies:

  - cognitive–behavioural therapy (CBT): the young person, sometimes with their family, learns to understand the links between their feelings and thoughts and how this affects their behaviour;
  - family-focused treatment (family therapy): the whole family can be helped to reduce stress, solve problems and communicate better.

- **Medication**

  Medication plays an important role in the treatment of bipolar disorder, especially if the episodes are severe. The choice of medication can depend on the type of episode (manic or depressive). Everyone is different, and so the type of medication that is recommended will also be different.

Medications can have mild, but also severe, side-effects. Your psychiatrist will be able to advise about what they are and what can be done to help. The risk of side-effects needs to be balanced against the risk of the damaging effects of the illness on a person's life.

Antipsychotic medications are usually prescribed for high/manic episodes, whereas antidepressant medications are used for the low/depressive episodes. You may also need medications called mood stabilisers (e.g. lithium) which help keep your mood stable both during and between episodes.

It is important that medications are not taken only when the problems are serious. If you have had more than one severe episode of illness, staying on medication is important to reduce the risk of further episodes. Medication may be needed for months or even years. Some people may, under medical supervision, be able to stop their medication when they have recovered and have felt well for a while.

You may need physical examination and tests (like a blood test) before starting or while you are on medication. It is important that if you are prescribed medication, you are regularly seen by your doctor or psychiatrist.

How long will I have the illness?

The high or low episodes can last from a few weeks to months. It is important to recognise that you are not alone and to keep up hope. Some people only ever experience one or two episodes, but for others the highs and lows can occur throughout their adult life. When this happens, it is important that you learn to live with the illness and manage it.

What can I do?

- The first step is recognising that something is different or that there is a problem. Other people are likely to have noticed that you seem different from your usual self, particularly those who live with you.
- Speak to people who know you well, such as family and friends.
- Seeking medical advice early on is very important. If the bipolar illness is identified and treated quickly, its harmful effects can be reduced.
- If you already have a diagnosis, try to understand your illness and problems as this can help you to take control and get help before it gets more difficult. This can mean steps like planning for a crisis and making choices about your career.
- Do things which help you to have good health, like having a balanced, healthy diet, doing some exercise, and getting a good night's sleep.
- Try to identify what makes you feel stressed and find ways of dealing with it.

How do I get help?

You may need to see your GP to talk about your concerns. They can then refer you to your local child and adolescent mental health service (CAMHS) which can offer more specialist help. If you have a school counsellor/nurse or learning mentor, they can also be a useful person to talk to and may also be able to refer you to the local CAMHS.

Rachel's story

'Rachel is a 15-year-old girl who has suffered episodes of depression in the past. Two months ago she started to talk very quickly and seemed to have lots of energy. She was excited about everything and was making all her friends laugh a lot.

Over a three-day period Rachel barely slept or ate, and started to say things that did not really make sense; for example, she told friends that she was a princess in Taiwan. She also started swearing and became extremely flirtatious which was out of character. She is quoted as saying, "I've never felt so great - I'm flying. I'm eleven on a scale of one to ten."

Rachel's parents were very worried and on the fourth night of her not sleeping, they took her to the local A&E department where she was seen by a psychiatrist who arranged for her to stay in hospital. A diagnosis of bipolar disorder was confirmed and treatment was given to bring Rachel's mood back to normal. She now has treatment to help prevent episodes of both depressed and abnormally high mood in the future.

She has been working with a community psychiatric nurse to improve her ability to recognise her own mood state and take measures to protect herself from further episodes.' ✪

Extract from The Young Mind: An Essential Guide to Mental Health for Young Adults, Parents and Teachers.

Recommended reading

Other factsheets in this series: Psychosis, CBT, Coping with stress, CAMHS

Rutter's Child and Adolescent Psychiatry (5th edn), edited by Sir Michael Rutter, Dorothy Bishop, Daniel Pine, et al. Published by Wiley–Blackwell (2008).

The Young Mind: An Essential Guide to Mental Health for Young Adults, Parents and Teachers, edited by Sue Bailey and Mike Shooter (2009) – an accessible, user-friendly handbook produced by the Royal College of Psychiatrists.

References

Fristad MA, Verducci JS, Walters K, et al. Impact of multifamily psychoeducational psychotherapy in treating children aged 8 to 12 years with mood disorders. *Arch Gen Psychiatry* 2009; 66: 1013–21.

Goodwin GM, Consensus Group of the British Association for Psychopharmacology. Evidence-based guidelines for treating bipolar disorder: revised second edition – recommendations from the British Association for Psychopharmacology. *J Psychopharmacol* 2009; 23: 346–88.

Leibenluft E, Dickstein DP. Bipolar disorder in children and adolescents. In *Rutter's Child and Adolescent Psychiatry* (5th edn) (eds M Rutter, D Bishop, D Pine, et al): 894–905. Wiley–Blackwell, 2008.

National Institute for Health and Clinical Excellence. *The Management of Bipolar Disorder in Adults, Children and Adolescents, in Primary and Secondary Care* (CG38). NICE, 2006.

Useful websites

- ⮑ **Bipolar UK**: www.bipolaruk.org.uk; helps people with bipolar disorder, their relatives, friends and others who care, and educates the public and caring professions about bipolar disorder. They produce a range of leaflets and support a network of self-help groups across the UK.
- ⮑ **Rethink Mental Illness**: www.rethink.org; a charity which helps people affected by a severe mental illness to recover a better quality of life. Their website has a section for young people.
- ⮑ **Sane**: www.sane.org.uk; a national charity which improves the quality of life for people affected by mental illness.
- ⮑ **Young Minds**: www.youngminds.org.uk; a charity committed to improving the emotional well-being and mental health of children and young people.

Notes

....

....

....

....

....

....

....

....

....

....

....

....

....

For a catalogue of public education materials or copies of our leaflets contact: Book Sales/Leaflets, The Royal College of Psychiatrists, 17 Belgrave Square, London SW1X 8PG. Email: leaflets@rcpsych.ac.uk, tel: 020 7235 2351 ext. 6146.

Revised by the Royal College of Psychiatrists' Child and Family Public Education Editorial Board. With grateful thanks to Very Important Kids (VIKs) from Young Minds for commenting on this factsheet and to Dr Sarah Bates for updating it. This leaflet reflects the best possible evidence at the time of writing.

2 Cannabis and mental health
Information for young people

This is one in a series of factsheets for young people, with practical, up-to-date information about mental health problems (emotional, behavioural and psychiatric disorders) that can affect children and young people.

This factsheet gives some basic information about cannabis and how it might affect your mental health.

Lots of young people want to know about drugs. Often, people around you are taking them, and you may wonder how it will make you feel. You may even feel under pressure to use drugs in order to fit in, or be 'cool'. You may have heard that cannabis is no worse than cigarettes, or that it is harmless.

What does it do to you?

When you smoke cannabis, the active compounds reach your brain quickly through your bloodstream. They then bind/stick to a special receptor in your brain. This causes your nerve cells to release different chemicals, and causes the effects that you feel. These effects can be enjoyable or unpleasant.

Often the bad effects take longer to appear than the pleasant ones.

- **Pleasant effects**: you may feel relaxed and talkative, and colours or music may seem more intense.

- **Unpleasant effects**: feeling sick/panicky, feeling paranoid or hearing voices, feeling depressed and unmotivated.

Unfortunately, some people can find cannabis addictive and so have trouble stopping use even when they are not enjoying it.

Louise's story

'When I was 16, I had my first joint. It was to help me with revising or for my exams. My friend told me that it would help me relax, and I could revise better. At first it worked, I felt calmer, more relaxed. But then I started forgetting things I'd revised and stressing myself out more. I started smoking more and more, and eventually I was relying on weed to cope. I started smoking more and more, every day, and it ended up being the only way that I could enjoy myself and have fun. My mum noticed that my eyes were always red, but just thought that I was ill. She took me to the doctor who tested my blood, and found out about my drug use. They got me help, and showed me other ways of getting rid of my stress. I ended up slowly cutting down on my cannabis use, and I have now stopped smoking completely.

When I look back, I realise how silly I was to start smoking so close to my exams. I had to retake a year of sixth form, and really regret developing such a strong addiction to cannabis. Although it seemed to help at the beginning, it did not help me in the long run. I now know that in order to do well in life, drugs are not the answer.' ✪

What is cannabis?

The cannabis plant is a member of the nettle family that has grown wild throughout the world for centuries. People have used it for lots of reasons, other than the popular relaxing effect.

It comes in two main forms:

- resin, which is a brown black lump also known as bhang, ganja or hashish
- herbal cannabis, which is made up of the dried leaves and flowering tops, and is known as grass, marijuana, spliff, weed, etc.

Skunk cannabis is made from a cannabis plant that has more active chemicals in it (THC), and the effect on your brain is stronger. Because 'street' cannabis varies so much in strength, you will not be able to tell exactly how it will make you feel at any particular time.

The effects of cannabis on your mental health

Using cannabis triggers mental health problems in people who seemed to be well before, or it can worsen any mental health problems you already have. Research has shown that people who are already at risk of developing mental health problems are more likely to start showing symptoms of mental illness if they use cannabis regularly. For example, if someone in your family has depression or schizophrenia, you are at higher risk of getting these illnesses when you use cannabis.

The younger you are when you start using it, the more you may be at risk. This is because your brain is still developing and can be more easily damaged by the active chemicals in cannabis.

If you stop using cannabis once you have started to show symptoms of mental illness, such as depression, paranoia or hearing voices, these symptoms may go away. However, not everyone will get better just by stopping smoking.

If you go on using cannabis, the symptoms can get worse. It can also make any treatment that your doctor might prescribe for you work less well. Your illness may come back more quickly, and more often if you continue to use cannabis once you get well again.

Some people with mental health problems find that using cannabis makes them feel a bit better for a while. Unfortunately, this does not last, and it does nothing to treat the illness. In fact, it may delay you from getting the help you need and the illness may get worse in the longer term.

What can you do?

If you are at all worried about the effect that cannabis might be having on your mental health, talk to somebody about it. This could be friends, family, or any professional such as:

- doctor or nurse
- teacher or school/college counsellor
- youth counsellor
- social worker.

There are lots of people who can help you decide whether you do have a problem and what you can do about it. However, if you don't talk about it, you are unlikely to get help.

Mental health problems generally do get better if you treat them quickly. In the meantime, there are several things you can do to help yourself:

- have a day without cannabis
- avoid bulk buying
- avoid people, places and activities that you associate with cannabis use
- do not use it if you are feeling sad or depressed
- STOP if you get hallucinations
- seek help.

Recommended reading

Other factsheets in this series: Worries and anxieties, Coping with stress, When bad things happen

Rutter's Child and Adolescent Psychiatry (5th edn), edited by Sir Michael Rutter, Dorothy Bishop, Daniel Pine, et al. Wiley–Blackwell (2008).

The Young Mind: An Essential Guide to Mental Health for Young Adults, Parents and Teachers, edited by Sue Bailey and Mike Shooter (2009) – an accessible, user-friendly handbook produced by the Royal College of Psychiatrists.

References

Di Forti M, Morgan C, Dazzan P, et al. High-potency cannabis and the risk of psychosis. *Br J Psychiatry* 2009; 195: 488–91.

Fergusson DM, Poulton R, Smith PF, et al. Cannabis and psychosis. *BMJ* 2006; 332:172–5.

Maddock C, Babbs M. Interventions for cannabis misuse. *Adv Psychiatr Treat* 2006; 12: 432–9.

Patton GC, Coffey C, Carlin, JB, et al. Cannabis use and mental health in young people: cohort study. *BMJ* 2002; 325: 1195–8.

Useful websites

Here are some websites which have more information about the effects of cannabis and other drugs on your mental health and what you can do.

- **City of London Substance Misuse Partnership**: www.cityoflondon.gov.uk/services/adult-health-wellbeing-and-social-care/drugs-and-alcohol/substance-misuse-partnership/Pages/Information-Leaflets.aspx; leaflets with useful information and harm minimisation advice on drugs and drug use.
- **Know Cannabis**: www.knowcannabis.org.uk; a website that can help you assess your cannabis use, its impact on your life and how to make changes if you want to.
- **Talk to Frank**: www.talktofrank.com; free and confidential drugs information and advice. Helpline: 0800 776600.
- **Young Minds**: www.youngminds.org.uk; a charity committed to improving the emotional well-being and mental health of children and young people.

Notes

....

....

For a catalogue of public education materials or copies of our leaflets contact: Book Sales/Leaflets, The Royal College of Psychiatrists, 17 Belgrave Square, London SW1X 8PG. Email: leaflets@rcpsych.ac.uk, tel: 020 7235 2351 ext. 6146.

Revised by the Royal College of Psychiatrists' Child and Family Public Education Editorial Board. With grateful thanks to Dr Nisha Shah. This leaflet reflects the best possible evidence at the time of writing.
The Royal College of Psychiatrists is a charity registered in England and Wales (228636) and in Scotland (SC038369).
© The Royal College of Psychiatrists 2013

3 Cognitive–behavioural therapy (CBT)
Information for young people

This is one in a series of factsheets for young people, with practical, up-to-date information about mental health problems (emotional, behavioural and psychiatric disorders) that can affect children and young people.

This factsheet explains what cognitive–behavioural therapy is, when it is used and how it can help you.

When is CBT used as treatment?

Cognitive–behavioural therapy is used to treat a wide range of mental health problems. In some conditions there is clear evidence of it being effective. These conditions include:

- low self-esteem
- depression
- anxiety problems
- obsessive–compulsive disorder (OCD)
- post-traumatic stress disorder (PTSD).

Cognitive–behavioural therapy can be used with medication and many people find this combination is better than medication alone.

How does it help?

Our thoughts and emotions often cause us problems. For example, think of a situation as below. The left-hand column illustrates how an unhelpful thought leads to feelings and behaviours different from the right-hand column. Here the same situation, with helpful thoughts, leads to a different outcome.

> **What is cognitive–behavioural therapy?**
>
> Cognitive–behavioural therapy (CBT) is a type of psychological treatment, also commonly known as a 'talking therapy'. It can help you understand how your problems began and what keeps them going.
>
> It works by helping you understand the links between:
>
> - what you think (your thoughts, beliefs and assumptions)
> - what you feel (your emotions)
> - what you do (your behaviour).

Situation: Your friend doesn't ring you	
Unhelpful thoughts: 'They don't like me'	*Helpful thoughts*: 'Something is wrong'
Feeling: You feel sad	*Feeling*: You are worried about your friend
Physical: You feel sick	*Physical*: You feel fine
Action: You don't go to your friend's party	*Action*: You ring – they had lost their mobile. You go to the party and enjoy yourself.

The key point is that sometimes our thoughts are unhelpful, and sometimes they are not accurate. This pattern of thinking can lead to many problems. Cognitive–behavioural therapy breaks these unhelpful patterns and helps you to feel more in control of your life.

What will CBT do for me?

Cognitive–behavioural therapy is not about thinking more positively! It helps improve the way you feel, think and what you do. It gives you skills for coping with your life. The goal of CBT is to help you learn a more balanced way of thinking, and to change any unhelpful patterns of thinking and behaving. This is important because sometimes, when you talk about things that are difficult, you may feel worse to begin with.

Cognitive–behavioural therapy teaches you skills:

- to overcome problematic thoughts, emotions and behaviour
- to find ways of overcoming negative thinking, challenging unhelpful and inaccurate thoughts or beliefs.

If I agree to take part in CBT, what will I have to do?

Initially, you may be seen by a therapist to make sure you can do the therapy (also called an 'assessment'). This usually means trying to understand your difficulties and agreeing what you wish to change in the present time. If you are offered CBT, you will be expected to meet with your therapist regularly (usually starting with once a week). The session can last up to an hour. To help your therapist to understand your difficulties, you will be asked to complete some questionnaires or worksheets. These may be repeated throughout your treatment. Your therapist will monitor how you are getting on.

The therapist will help you understand your problems and teach you ways of dealing with them. You will be expected to practise them outside of your therapy (e.g. at school or college or at home). This means that tasks or homework will be set at the end of the meeting. You may be given worksheets to help remind you of what you need to do.

Why do I have to do tasks between sessions?

You cannot learn to ride a bike by reading a book. Any skill you want to learn requires practice, and CBT requires this too.

It is important to practise the CBT skills you are taught:

- to be sure that you understand them
- to check that you can use them when you need to (e.g. when you are feeling upset about something)
- so that any problems you may have in using these skills can be worked on in your therapy.

It is not always easy to learn new skills, so you will need lots of support from your therapist, as well as your family and carers.

How many sessions of CBT will I be expected to attend?

For more simple problems, six to ten sessions can be enough to help you overcome your difficulties. You may be offered more sessions if you have more severe problems. Your difficulties will be regularly monitored by your therapist. It may seem like hard work at times, but by attending sessions and learning new ways of coping, you will be equipping yourself with valuable life skills.

> **Jane, 14, talks about having CBT**
>
> 'I was falling behind in my schoolwork and finding it hard to concentrate at school. I was becoming really quiet and my mates were wondering what was happening as I didn't want to go out anymore. I thought that no one liked me. I just couldn't be bothered doing anything.
>
> At the time I thought my Mum was nagging at me to do more things, as she noticed that I was spending more time in my room. I did realise that Mum was trying to help and she took me to a psychiatrist who was nice and listened to what I was going through. He mentioned a therapy called CBT and said that it would help me.
>
> I met with my therapist regularly over a few months and it was really practical. It was different from anything I had done before – it helped me to think about the thoughts and feelings I was having at the time. I learnt why I was having a hard time and learnt some ways of coping better. I started doing things differently. Something that I really liked was how the therapist and I set a plan of what we would be talking about together. I started doing things again that I had been avoiding. I am able to focus at school again and I am seeing friends. Plus, I find that exercise helps me to deal with stress and unhappy feelings.' ✪

Where and how can I get this type of treatment?

Cognitive–behavioural therapy can be offered by trained therapists at child and adolescent mental health services (CAMHS). Sometimes, when your problems are not severe, you may be able to receive help from trained staff in school (e.g. special educational needs coordinating officer (SENCO)/school nurse), counsellors or voluntary agencies.

For older adolescents and adults, there also is a computerised package of treatment available for specific conditions (e.g. depression). You may also find reading self-help books useful.

Recommended reading

Other factsheets in this series: Coping with stress, CAMHS

Rutter's Child and Adolescent Psychiatry (5th edn), edited by Sir Michael Rutter, Dorothy Bishop, Daniel Pine, et al. Wiley–Blackwell (2008).

The Young Mind: An Essential Guide to Mental Health for Young Adults, Parents and Teachers, edited by Sue Bailey and Mike Shooter (2009) – an accessible, user-friendly handbook produced by the Royal College of Psychiatrists.

References

National Institute for Health and Clinical Health and Excellence. *Depression in Children and Young People* (CG28). NICE, 2005.

Williams C. Therapies, treatments and medication: cognitive behavioural therapy. In *The Mind: A User's Guide* (ed R Persaud): 427–437. Bantam Press, 2007.

Useful websites

- **British Association for Behavioural and Cognitive Psychotherapies**: www.babcp.com; a UK charity for people involved in the practice and theory of behavioural and cognitive psychotherapy. It gives information on therapy including signposting to self-help materials and therapists.
- **Cognitive Behaviour Therapy Self-Help Resources**: www.getselfhelp.co.uk; CBT self-help information, resources and therapy worksheets.
- **Young Minds**: www.youngminds.org.uk; a charity committed to improving the emotional well-being and mental health of children and young people.
- **Youth2Youth**: www.youth2youth.co.uk; UK's national young person's helpline run by young people for young people. Tel. 020 8896 3675.

Notes

For a catalogue of public education materials or copies of our leaflets contact: Book Sales/Leaflets, The Royal College of Psychiatrists, 17 Belgrave Square, London SW1X 8PG. Email: leaflets@rcpsych.ac.uk, tel: 020 7235 2351 ext. 6146.

Revised by the Royal College of Psychiatrists' Child and Family Public Education Editorial Board. With grateful thanks to Dr Fareeha Amber Sadiq. This leaflet reflects the best possible evidence at the time of writing.

4 Coping with stress
Information for young people

This is one in a series of factsheets for young people, with practical, up-to-date information about mental health problems (emotional, behavioural and psychiatric disorders) that can affect children and young people.

This factsheet looks at what stress is, what causes it and how it might feel to be suffering from stress. It also gives some practical advice about how to cope with different types of stress.

What causes stress?

There are many reasons why you might feel stressed, for example:

- schoolwork piling up
- preparing for exams
- being teased or bullied at school
- arguing with parents, brothers or sisters, or friends.

Stress can be even worse if your family is breaking up, someone close to you is ill or dies, or if you are being physically or sexually abused.

People vary in the amount that they get stressed by things – you may find that you get very stressed out by exams, but your friends don't seem bothered.

Positive events can also be stressful. For example, starting a new college or going to university. Many people need a little bit of stress to give them the 'get up and go' to do things that are important to them.

What are the effects of stress?

Stress can affect different people in different ways. Stress can affect your body and your feelings. Some of the effects are listed below.

Effects of stress on your body:

- feeling tired
- having difficulty sleeping
- going off your food
- stomach aches
- headaches
- aches and pains in your neck and shoulders.

Effects of stress on your feelings:

- feeling sad
- being irritable, losing your temper easily
- finding it hard to keep your mind on schoolwork.

How do I cope with stress?

There are several things that you can do to help yourself cope.

- Don't suffer in silence! Feeling alone makes stress harder to deal with.
- Talking to somebody you trust can really help you to deal with stress and to work out how to tackle the problems that are causing it.
- Make a list of all the things in your life that are making you feel stressed – write them down on a piece of paper. Then take each one in turn and list all the things you could do to tackle it. This can help you sort things out in your head. Problems look easier to deal with one at a time than in a big jumble in your head.

What is stress?

People get stressed when they feel like the demands or pressures on them are more than what they can cope with.

Everyone feels stressed at times. You may feel under pressure, worried, tense, upset, sad and angry – or maybe a mixture of uncomfortable feelings. These feelings can be entirely normal, but sometimes stress can get too much and can even trigger a mental illness.

Sometimes people try to 'block out' stress by using drugs or alcohol. This makes things worse in the long run. It is important to get help if stress is getting too much or you are using drugs or alcohol to try to cope.

- Take a break – do something that you really enjoy.
- Do something relaxing, for example, take a hot bath or watch a film.
- Do some exercise. This produces chemicals in your body called endorphins which make you feel good.

When to get help?

Sometimes stress gets on top of you, especially when the situation causing the stress goes on and on and the problems just seem to keep building up. You can feel trapped, as if there is no way out and no solution to your problems. If you feel like this, it is important to get help.

Signs that stress is getting too much and that you should get help:

- you feel that stress is affecting your health
- you feel so desperate that you think about stopping school, running away or harming yourself
- you feel low, sad, tearful, or that life is not worth living
- you lose your appetite and find it difficult to sleep
- you have worries, feelings and thoughts that are hard to talk about because you feel people won't understand you or will think you are 'weird'
- you hear voices telling you what to do, or making you behave strangely
- you are using drugs or alcohol to block out stress.

Who can help?

It is important that you talk to someone you trust and who can help you, for example:

- a close friend
- parents, a family member or family friend
- a school nurse, teacher or school counsellor
- a social worker or youth counsellor
- a priest, someone from your church or temple.

Some people may find it easier to talk to somebody on the phone. See the useful websites box at the end of this factsheet for details of confidential advice lines.

Your GP or another professional can refer you to your local child and adolescent mental health service (CAMHS).

Chloe's story (16)

'It started a few months ago, during year 11. I had a lot of work to do because it was my GCSE year but I was off for 2 weeks in April because I had tonsillitis and I needed an operation. When I went back to school, I had missed tons of work and I was given extra homework to do to catch up. I tried really hard to get this done on top of my coursework, but I just got more and more behind. I started to think I'd never be able to catch up and I thought I'd fail all my GCSEs. It got to the point where I couldn't sleep because I was worrying too much. Although I was spending more and more time doing homework, I couldn't actually concentrate on it because I just kept thinking about how much I had to do. I was really snappy and horrible to my family and I had stopped seeing my friends.

I didn't want to get any help because I thought I'd look stupid, but my Mum dragged me to see my head of year. I'm glad my Mum did that because she was really understanding about the mess I had got in and she helped me to sort it out. She spoke to my class teachers and they agreed that I didn't need to do all of the outstanding work, just the most important bits. Two of my teachers spent some time with me after school, going through some bits of my courses I hadn't understood properly. I was given some time out of lessons to catch up on my coursework.

Within a couple of weeks I had caught up and I was feeling much better because I was sleeping properly and seeing friends again. I got good grades in my GCSEs and I'm going to college in September.' ✪

Recommended reading

Other factsheets in this series: Exercise and mental health, When bad things happen, CAMHS

Rays of Calm: Relaxation for Teenagers, by Christiane Kerr. This is a CD from the 'Calm for Kids' range created for teenagers. It talks through various relaxation techniques and visualisations designed to promote a sense of calm and well-being and to help teenagers deal with stress.

The Young Mind: An Essential Guide to Mental Health for Young Adults, Parents and Teachers, edited by Sue Bailey and Mike Shooter (2009) – an accessible, user-friendly handbook produced by the Royal College of Psychiatrists.

References

Gelder M, Harrison P, Cowen P. *Shorter Oxford Textbook of Psychiatry* (5th edn) Oxford University Press, 2006.

Kraag G, Van Breukelen GJ, Kok G, et al. 'Learn Young, Learn Fair', a stress management program for fifth and sixth graders: longitudinal results from an experimental study. *J Child Psychology Psychiatry* 2009; 50: 1185–95.

Rutter M, Bishop D, Pine D, et al (eds) *Rutter's Child and Adolescent Psychiatry* (5th edn). Wiley–Blackwell, 2008.

Seiffge-Krenke I, Aunola K, Nurmi JE. Changes in stress perception and coping during adolescence: the role of situational and personal factors. *Child Dev* 2009; 80: 259–79.

Useful websites

- **ChildLine**: www.childline.org.uk; a free and confidential telephone service for children. You can also get in touch by email or by confidential live one-to-one chat. Helpline: 0800 1111.
- **Samaritans**: www.samaritans.org; a 24-hour service offering confidential emotional support to anyone who is in crisis. Helpline 08457 909090 (UK), 1850 609090 (Ireland), email: jo@samaritans.org.
- **Talk to Frank**: www.talktofrank.com;free and confidential drugs information and advice. Helpline: 0800 776600.
- **Teenage Health Freak**: www.teenagehealthfreak.org; accurate and reliable health information for teenagers.
- **Young Minds**: www.youngminds.org.uk; a charity committed to improving the emotional well-being and mental health of children and young people.
- **Youth Access**: www.youthaccess.org.uk; information, advice and counselling throughout the UK.

Notes

For a catalogue of public education materials or copies of our leaflets contact: Book Sales/Leaflets, The Royal College of Psychiatrists, 17 Belgrave Square, London SW1X 8PG. Email: leaflets@rcpsych.ac.uk, tel: 020 7235 2351 ext. 6146.

Revised by the Royal College of Psychiatrists' Child and Family Public Education Editorial Board. With grateful thanks to Dr Sarah Bates. This leaflet reflects the best possible evidence at the time of writing.

5 Depression
Information for young people

This is one in a series of factsheets for young people, with practical, up-to-date information about mental health problems (emotional, behavioural and psychiatric disorders) that can affect children and young people.

This factsheet looks at how to recognise depression and what you can do to help yourself or someone else who has depression.

How common is depression?

Depression usually starts in your teenage years, more commonly as you near adulthood. It is less common in children under 12 years old. It can affect anybody, although it is more common in girls than in boys.

How do I know if I have it?

Some of the signs that you may have depression are:

- being moody and irritable, easily upset, 'ratty' or tearful
- becoming withdrawn, avoiding friends, family and regular activities
- feeling guilty or bad, being self-critical and self-blaming, hating yourself
- feeling unhappy, miserable and lonely a lot of the time
- feeling hopeless and wanting to die
- finding it difficult to concentrate
- not looking after your personal appearance
- changes in sleep pattern: sleeping too little or too much
- feeling tired
- not interested in eating, eating little or too much
- suffering aches and pains, such as headaches or stomach aches
- feeling you are not good-looking.

If you have all or most of these signs, and have had them over a long period of time, it may mean that you have depression. You may find it very difficult to talk about how you are feeling.

> ### What is depression?
>
> Most people, children as well as adults, feel low or 'blue' occasionally. Feeling sad is a normal reaction to experiences that are stressful or upsetting. However, when these feelings go on and on, take over your usual self and interfere with your whole life, it can become an illness. This illness is called 'depression'.

What causes depression?

There is no specific cause of depression. It is usually caused by a mixture of things, rather than any one thing alone.

- Events or personal experiences can be a trigger. These include family breakdown, the death or loss of someone you love, neglect, abuse, bullying and physical illness.
- Depression can start if too many changes happen in your life too quickly.
- You are more likely to have depression if you are under a lot of stress and have no one to share your worries with.
- Depression may run in families and can be more common if you already suffer from physical illness or difficulties. Depression seems to be linked with chemical changes in the part of the brain that controls mood.

What can I do if I am feeling low?

You can try a few things to see if it helps you feel better. Simply talking to someone you trust and who you feel understands can lighten the burden. It can also make it easier to work out practical solutions to problems. For example, if you feel unable to do your homework, letting your family and teachers know can be helpful for you to get some support to complete your work.

Sarah, 16, talks about her depression

'I was 15. They took me to see the doctor because they thought I was a bit down and I had started cutting. I hadn't noticed much, cutting made me feel better and I just felt they were having a bit of a go really. It was only when I started to talk more that I realised how much I had changed, I used to be happy, not all the time, but I couldn't now – not like I used to.

I was falling out with my teachers - they said I wasn't getting on with work and it made me cross. I was trying but I just couldn't get on with it, not like I did in year 8 and 9. The doctor said it could be my concentration. I hadn't thought of that, I just thought I was thick. Then when he asked about other things, I started to see. I couldn't sleep properly and didn't feel like going out to play football anymore. I said it was just boring, but as I started to feel better, I did play again and I think saying it was boring was all part of my depression. That was the same with my family, I mean you don't get on all time do you and they are still a pain sometimes now, but when I was depressed it was like we were always arguing, I just couldn't talk to them and they just wound me up. It wasn't till they talked to me and things started to change, that was when I looked back and realised how depressed I was.' ✪

Here are some things to try:

- talk to someone whom you trust and who can help
- try to do some physical activity and eat healthy food
- try to keep yourself occupied by doing activities, even if you feel you do not really enjoy them
- try not to stay all alone in your room, especially during the day
- don't overstress yourself, and allow for fun and leisure time.

How parents/family and teachers can help?

When you have depression, you may feel ashamed and guilty about the way you are. You may worry about upsetting others, especially family, or being told you are making it up or blamed it is your fault by telling them how you feel. It can also be very hard to put your feelings into words. However, many young people in a similar situation feel a sense of relief at being understood once they have talked about it. Letting others know about how you feel is important for getting the right help and support.

When should I get more help?

Many young people will get better on their own with support and understanding. If the depression is dragging on and causing serious difficulties, it is important to seek treatment. Sometimes when you are feeling low, you may try to use drugs or alcohol to forget your feelings. You may see no hope and feel like running away from it all. Doing this only makes the situation worse. When this happens it is important that you let others know and get help.

Where can I get help?

Your GP, or sometimes school nurse, will be able to advise you about what help is available and to arrange a referral to the local child and adolescent mental health service (CAMHS). They will see you and your family and discuss the right treatment for you.

How is depression treated?

When the depression is not very bad, which means you are still able to do your daily activities like going to school, you may find psychological therapies, also called talking therapies, helpful. Cognitive–behavioural therapy (CBT) is one of these and it is effective for treating depression.

Other talking therapies can also be helpful, for example family therapy and interpersonal therapy, both of which may be available from your CAMHS.

When your depression is severe and has been going on for a long time, you may find it difficult to even talk about it. In this situation, medications can help to lift your mood. Medications called antidepressants are usually used for depression. They need to be prescribed by specialist child and adolescent psychiatrists (CAMHS) after a careful assessment. If you are given medication, you may need a physical health check-up beforehand, and then you will need regular check-ups once you have started on the medication.

Medications are usually given for a few months, and sometimes may need to be taken for a longer time. It is important that you take your medication the way it has been prescribed for you (i.e. the right dose and timing).

Remember that you are not alone – depression is a common problem and can be overcome.

Recommended reading

Other factsheets in this series: CBT, When bad things happen, CAMHS

Changing Minds. Mental Health: What it is, What to do, Where to go? This is a CD produced by the Royal College of Psychiatrists for 13- to 17-year-olds. It talks about addiction, stress, eating disorders, depression, schizophrenia and self-harm.

The Young Mind: An Essential Guide to Mental Health for Young Adults, Parents and Teachers, edited by Sue Bailey and Mike Shooter (2009) – an accessible, user-friendly handbook produced by the Royal College of Psychiatrists.

References

National Institute for Health and Clinical Health and Excellence. *Depression in Children and Young People* (CG28). NICE, 2005.

Rutter M, Bishop D, Pine D, et al (eds) *Rutter's Child and Adolescent Psychiatry* (5th edn). Wiley–Blackwell, 2008.

Useful websites

- **Campaign Against Living Miserably (CALM)**: www.thecalmzone.net; a campaign and charity targeting young men, with a helpline, magazine and online community, but CALM listens to anyone who needs help or support.
- **ChildLine**: www.childline.org.uk; free and confidential service for children. Helpline 0800 1111.
- **Depression Alliance**: www.depressionalliance.org; help and information about depression, depression symptoms and self-help groups.
- **Rethink**: www.rethink.org; mental health charity helping people with mental health problems. Their website has a section for young people.
- **YoungMinds**: www.youngminds.org.uk; provides information and advice on child mental health issues.

Notes

....
....
....
....
....
....
....
....
....

For a catalogue of public education materials or copies of our leaflets contact: Book Sales/Leaflets, The Royal College of Psychiatrists, 17 Belgrave Square, London SW1X 8PG. Email: leaflets@rcpsych.ac.uk, tel: 020 7235 2351 ext. 6146.

Revised by the Royal College of Psychiatrists' Child and Family Public Education Editorial Board. With grateful thanks to Dr Fareeha Amber Sadiq. This leaflet reflects the best possible evidence at the time of writing.

6 Drugs and alcohol
Information for young people

This is one in a series of factsheets for young people, with practical, up-to-date information about mental health problems (emotional, behavioural and psychiatric disorders) that can affect children and young people.

This factsheet aims to point out the problems with misusing drugs and alcohol, and gives you some ideas about how to avoid them.

What are the commonly used drugs?

Society's favourite drugs are alcohol and tobacco. They are both very addictive and are misused by millions of people. There are many other drugs which are addictive. Some of these are 'legal' and others 'illegal'.

Some legal substances, such as petrol and glue, if misused, can be very harmful. Even medicines such as painkillers and certain drugs for sleep problems can be addictive, particularly if they are not used in the way they were prescribed. The obviously illegal drugs are things like cannabis (hash), speed (amphetamines), ecstasy ('E'), cocaine and heroin.

For more detailed information on drugs and their effects, see the websites listed at the end.

What is addiction?

Lots of young people want to know about drugs and alcohol. It is important to know that despite one's willpower, it is very easy to end up finding that you have a problem. You may initially think that you have your drug or alcohol use 'under control', however, these things can be very addictive and may soon start to control you.

Why do people take drugs or alcohol?

People may do this for many reasons:

- they may worry that if they don't take drugs, they will be seen as 'uncool' and won't fit in
- they may just want to experiment
- they find that taking a particular drug makes them feel confident and may help them to face a difficult situation
- if they are unhappy, stressed or lonely, they are more likely to turn to drugs to forget their problems.

What leads to problems with drugs and alcohol?

Problems can happen for different reasons.

- Drugs can make you feel good for a while. Just experimenting with a drug may make you want to try again … and again.
- If you take drugs or alcohol to help cope with a situation or a feeling, after a while you may need the drug to face that situation or feeling every time.
- If you find that you are using a drug or alcohol more and more often, be careful as this is the first step to becoming dependent on it.
- If you hang out with people who use a lot of drugs or drink heavily, you probably will too.

What are the dangers of taking drugs and alcohol?

Drugs and alcohol damage your health. Here are some basic facts.

- It is dangerous to mix drugs and alcohol. They each may increase the effects of the other substance, e.g. ecstasy and alcohol can lead to dehydration (overheating) and cause coma and death.
- You cannot know for sure what is in the drug you buy – it might not contain what the dealer says. Some dealers might mix it with other substances, or you may get a higher dose of a drug than you are used to which can be fatal.
- Sharing needles or other equipment can spread serious infections such as HIV and hepatitis.
- Accidents, arguments and fights are more likely after drinking and drug use.
- Using drugs can lead to serious mental illness, such as psychosis or depression, and to health problems and overdoses.

> **Johnny, 14, talks about his using drugs**
>
> 'I was 10 years old when my friend gave me some weed to try. It felt a bit weird, I didn't really like it but I still did it with my friends. It was just the "in" thing. I am not really sure when it all changed. I started thinking of ways of getting money or asking someone for it. I tried quite a few things. On Fridays and weekends I would have a few rounds of drink like vodka and even mix it with stuff. I smoked and had a couple of joints worth about 5–10 quid every day.
>
> My family did not really bother… at least not until now. Dad was too busy working shifts. Mum was tired looking after three of us on her own. I was always the black sheep. Jack and Lucy were the best kids in town, never in trouble, good grades… too perfect. So they never noticed until Jack saw me bunking off school and later having bruises after I had a fight after drinking. He told my parents.
>
> I was angry at first, told them it was all a lie and then that it was their fault. For months we had rows, I stayed with my nan. My drug counsellor was very patient with me. He explained to me about the effects drugs could have on me. I wish I had known about it before. He believed in me, did not give up… I could not let him down. I can talk more easily to my dad now… after years I feel he is really there. It is still difficult, but I am trying to study. I really enjoy the bricklaying experience. I have made new friends… friends who don't do drugs. It keeps me safe and happy.' ✪

How do I know when I am hooked?

The most common sign that you have a drug or alcohol problem is when you feel you no longer have a choice. You find yourself having to take the drug more and more to get the same effect. You may find it difficult to cope without it. You may say 'It's not that I need it', but find it is a habit that you are unable to give up.

Read and answer the questions below honestly.

- Do you think about drugs or alcohol every day?
- Is it hard to say 'no' when drugs or alcohol are offered?
- Would you drink/take drugs when you are alone?
- Does taking drugs/alcohol get in the way of the rest of your life?

If the answer to any of these questions is 'yes', you may be hooked.

What do I do if someone offers me drugs or alcohol?

It is sometimes difficult to say 'no'. You need to first be aware of what you are going to take and what it can do to you. Think before you answer: for example, you may say 'I have had it before and I don't like it'. Whatever you say, say it confidently and stick to it.

You may also find other ways – you have to go somewhere else, do something else you enjoy like sports, drama, etc. This makes it easier for you to leave and avoid getting into trouble with drugs or alcohol.

If you do take something, remember what the safe limits are for you. Think ahead, keep a watch on how much you take, and have a plan to stop or leave the situation.

What do I do if my friend or someone I know needs help?

It can be very difficult to see someone you like or care for having a drug or alcohol problem. You may try to tell them to stop, or suggest that they leave when they seem to be taking more than they should. Don't try talking to them when they are drunk or have taken a lot of drugs – it's best to speak to them the next day. You may suggest that they should get help (see websites listed at the end of this factsheet).

In an emergency, such as if your friend falls unconscious or hurts themselves, don't hesitate to call an ambulance for help.

Remember: you are not responsible for what your friend does. Take care of yourself, speak to others, for instance your family or a teacher you can trust and talk to.

Where can I get help?

There are different ways of getting help. It is good to first talk to someone you trust:

- a close friend
- your parents or a family member
- a family friend
- a school nurse
- a social worker
- a teacher/school counsellor.

Michelle, mum, talks about Johnny's drug use

'Johnny was always the boisterous one with a short fuse. So unlike his brother Jack and sister Lucy. He was good with doing things like making and fixing stuff, but not very good in English or other subjects. I thought he was more like his dad, Jake. Jake was away most of the time working as a truck driver. It was like being a single parent with three kids. I looked after the home, cooked, fed the kids and cleaned the house. But maybe I never spent much time with the kids. They were all good so I never really thought about it. Not until the day Jack came and told us about Johnny missing school and having bruises all over. I don't know how I missed it…there were some signs but I had just thought it was him being a teenager. Johnny's clothes were smelly, he used to come home really late at weekends and he did not look healthy.

He did not even eat much and only had coffee in the morning. It was like walking on fire when we first asked Johnny…I thought his life was over. I cried, felt guilty. The drug counsellor told us all about drugs, how we could help. Somehow I felt there was a ray of hope. It has been a long, rocky road but I feel stronger. Johnny is enjoying his vocational courses. We make sure we spend time as a family, go out, even though we can't afford much.

I wish I had known about these things before…maybe a parents' evening in school would've helped.' ✪

You may even like to speak to a professional, for example your GP or practice nurse, a local drug project or child and adolescent mental health service (CAMHS). They can refer you on to the relevant services, and will be able to offer you advice and support.

You can find useful contacts in your local area telephone book or on the local council website, or you can ask for the address from your health centre.

Recommended reading

Other factsheets in this series: CAMHS

The Young Mind: An Essential Guide to Mental Health for Young Adults, Parents and Teachers, edited by Sue Bailey and Mike Shooter (2009) – an accessible, user-friendly handbook produced by the Royal College of Psychiatrists.

References

National Institute for Health and Clinical Excellence. *Alcohol-Use Disorders: Diagnosis, Assessment and Management of Harmful Drinking and Alcohol Dependence* (CG115). NICE, 2011.

National Institute for Health and Clinical Excellence. *Drug Misuse: Psychosocial Interventions and Opioid Detoxification. Understanding NICE Guidance* (CG51). NICE, 2007.

Useful websites

Most of the websites below offer telephone advice or email contact.

⮑ **Drinkaware**: www.drinkaware.co.uk; information to make informed decisions about the effects of alcohol on your life.

⮑ **NHS Direct**: www.nhsdirect.nhs.uk; help and advice on any aspect of health and drug and alcohol use. Tel: 0845 4647.

⮑ **Smokefree**: http://smokefree.nhs.uk; an NHS smoking helpline. Tel: 0800 022 43 32.

⮑ **Talk to Frank**: www.talktofrank.com; free and confidential drugs information and advice line. Helpline: 0800 776600.

Notes

....

....

....

....

....

For a catalogue of public education materials or copies of our leaflets contact: Book Sales/Leaflets, The Royal College of Psychiatrists, 17 Belgrave Square, London SW1X 8PG. Email: leaflets@rcpsych.ac.uk, tel: 020 7235 2351 ext. 6146.

Revised by the Royal College of Psychiatrists' Child and Family Public Education Editorial Board. With grateful thanks to Dr Vasu Balaguru. This leaflet reflects the best possible evidence at the time of writing.
The Royal College of Psychiatrists is a charity registered in England and Wales (228636) and in Scotland (SC038369). © The Royal College of Psychiatrists 2013

7 Exercise and mental health
Information for young people

This is one in a series of factsheets for young people, with practical, up-to-date information about mental health problems (emotional, behavioural and psychiatric disorders) that can affect children and young people.

This factsheet explains the link between physical activity and mental health and offers some suggestions about getting started.

This factsheet is for young people who want to know:

- how being active can make you feel better
- how exercise can help depression and anxiety
- how active you need to be to feel better.

Why do exercise?

Exercise keeps our heart, body and mind healthy. There is evidence that exercise can help in depression, anxiety and even protects you from stress. To work properly, your body needs regular exercise.

Regular activity helps you to:
- feel good about yourself
- concentrate better
- sleep better
- have a positive outlook on life
- keep a healthy weight
- build healthy bones, muscles and joints.

Most of us feel good when we are active. So, don't worry about not doing enough – get started by building a bit of physical activity into your daily life now. Even a small change can get your heart healthier and make you feel happier.

Why does exercise make me feel better?

When you exercise, 'feel-good' chemicals called endorphins are released in your brain. Exercise also affects chemicals called dopamine and serotonin which are related to depression and anxiety. It can help brain cells to grow. In your body, regular exercise makes your heart, muscles and bones stronger and makes them work better.

Activity can help you feel more in control which helps when you are worried or stressed. You can even make new friends and have fun when you exercise with other people.

How much activity is enough for me?

Any activity is good. You should try to do some activity every day. Regular exercise for about 40 minutes which gets you out of breath, five times a week, will have the best results on your body and mood.

What is exercise?

Anything that gets your body active and makes you a bit out of breath is exercise. It might be sports such as football or netball, playing with friends or part of your everyday life, like a brisk walk to school.

Sarah, 15

'It's been a tough time. We had family problems and then I had exams on top. I started to get really stressed out, couldn't relax at night or concentrate at school. Sometimes I found myself just bursting into tears. I talked to my PE teacher at school who's really nice and suggested I take up running, which helped me to get some space for myself. I've really improved in how far I can go, but mostly I run because I enjoy it. It's given me my energy back. My sleep has got better and I don't feel so depressed anymore. A friend has asked if she can run with me sometimes. I'm kind of ready for that now.' ✪

What kind of exercise can I do?

You choose! Don't worry if you have never done it before or if you don't like sports. Exercise does not have to be about running around a track or going to a gym. It can be just about being more active each day.

There might be easy ways to get more active like getting off the bus and walking, taking the stairs instead of a lift or taking your dog for a walk. It might be active sports like football, netball, hockey or rugby, or you might prefer something less competitive like walking, jogging or rock climbing.

If you like something relaxing, then walking listening to music on earphones or doing yoga might suit you more. Have a look around and find something you think you'll enjoy.

What do I need to do to exercise healthily?

- Making the start is the first step.
- Start gently, especially if you have not done exercise for a long time. If you have physical health problems, do check with your doctor or specialist how much you can do and what best to avoid.
- Don't overdo it, even if you are very fit. Too much exercise or exercising too intensely will make you feel worse. Even Olympic athletes have to make sure they do not overstrain themselves.
- You may need to watch your diet. Make sure you are eating healthily, especially breakfast, and avoid too much tea, coffee or energy drinks.
- Watch your weight. Usually exercise helps us keep to a healthy weight, but sometimes it can get out of control. If your weight goes down too much it can cause problems.
- Avoid exercising too late in the day because it can make it hard to switch off and go to sleep.
- Finally, enjoy it. If you find it's making you anxious or unhappy, then speak to someone or check out the websites mentioned overleaf to find something that works better for you.

> **Tom, 13**
>
> 'We moved house last year and I started at a new school. It wasn't easy to make friends at first and I got picked on a bit. School went right downhill and I got into a few fights. One of the teaching assistants told me about a football team near where I live. I've met other young people and made some friends. My confidence has got better and I get less angry now. I go to training every week and last week I got the winning goal!' ✪

Getting down to it

The most important thing is to make a start. This might mean getting help and support from your friends, family, teacher, school or health professional such as a nurse. Making a plan to go with someone else can help you to keep going. Going to an exercise class or gym can boost your motivation.

Some people find using an exercise diary or timetable helpful. Writing the goals can make them easier to remember. Try to keep it simple and set a plan you can do for a few weeks. See how you do before you set the next target. It is important that you have fun. If you are finding it hard, boring or if it makes you feel worse, then think again, ask for help or try something new.

Nobody is perfect. You can have times when you find exercising difficult or stop doing it. Don't worry about it. Tomorrow is another day and you can start again. If you need to, talk to someone or ask for help.

Recommended reading

Other factsheets in this series: Coping with stress, Depression

Rutter's Child and Adolescent Psychiatry (5th edn), edited by Sir Michael Rutter, Dorothy Bishop, Daniel Pine, et al. Wiley–Blackwell, 2008.

The Young Mind: An Essential Guide to Mental Health for Young Adults, Parents and Teachers, edited by Sue Bailey and Mike Shooter (2009) – an accessible, user-friendly handbook produced by the Royal College of Psychiatrists.

References

Department of Health. *Start Active, Stay Active: A Report on Physical Activity for Health from the Four Home Countries' Chief Medical Officers.* Department of Health, 2011.

González-Gross M, Gómez-Lorente JJ, Valtueña J, et al. The 'healthy lifestyle guide pyramid' for children and adolescents. *Nutr Hosp* 2008; 23: 159–68.

Larun L, Nordheim LV, Ekeland E, et al. Exercise in prevention and treatment of anxiety and depression among children and young people. *Cochrane Database Syst Rev* 2009; 3: CD004691.

National Institute for Health and Clinical Excellence. *Depression: The Treatment and Management of Depression in Adults (Update) (CG90).* NICE, 2009.

Taylor AH, Faulkner G. Inaugural editorial. *Ment Health Phys Activity* 2008; 1: 1–8.

Useful websites

⟳ **Active Places**: www.activeplaces.com; this website allows you to search for sports facilities anywhere in England. You can browse an interactive map of the country, search for facilities in your local area, or use the name and address of a specific facility to find out more information.

⟳ **English Federation of Disability Sport**: www.efds.co.uk; organisation that supports and promotes sport for people with disabilities.

⟳ **Sustrans**: www.sustrans.co.uk; provides advice on cycling opportunities locally and further afield, including the National Cycle Network.

Notes

For a catalogue of public education materials or copies of our leaflets contact: Book Sales/Leaflets, The Royal College of Psychiatrists, 17 Belgrave Square, London SW1X 8PG. Email: leaflets@rcpsych.ac.uk, tel: 020 7235 2351 ext. 6146.

Revised by the Royal College of Psychiatrists' Child and Family Public Education Editorial Board. With grateful thanks to Dr Fareeha Amber Sadiq. This leaflet reflects the best possible evidence at the time of writing.

8 Mental illness in a parent
Information for young people

This is one in a series of factsheets for young people, with practical, up-to-date information about mental health problems (emotional, behavioural and psychiatric disorders) that can affect children and young people.

This factsheet is to help you answer some of the many questions you may have if you live with or have a parent with a mental illness. It explains what mental illness is, why it happens and what to do.

Why is it difficult when a parent has a mental illness?

Illness in someone you live with, especially a parent, is always difficult because the person who is there to look after you suddenly can't do it. Instead you may have to be the 'carer', which means you are the one who does the looking after.

With any illness everyday activities can be very difficult, but when a parent has a mental illness everything can be even more confusing because:

- your parent(s) may not look ill or stay in bed, but they might just behave and be different
- they may think and feel differently about things than they did before or compared with how other people think and feel.

When your parent is unwell, it can start affecting your everyday life, like having meals or going to school. Many children start thinking and blaming themselves for perhaps doing something wrong, worrying unnecessarily that they may have been naughty and somehow caused the illness. These thoughts are quite common among children and young people in these difficult situations – but of course these worries are not true.

What are the different types of mental illness?

There are various types of mental illness and various terms are used to describe them. Below we mention a few. **Remember, every illness is different and it can affect people in different ways.**

- When a person has **depression** they appear sad and/or tearful. They don't seem to enjoy anything, and find that they can't sleep or eat properly.
- When a person suffers from **anxiety** they may worry so much that they find it difficult to even go out. They may worry that bad things will happen.
- When a person has **obsessive–compulsive disorder** (commonly referred to as OCD), they can have worrying thoughts about keeping everything in order and having to do things in a very special way or performing 'rituals', such as repeatedly washing their hands or checking the doors.
- When a person has **psychosis** they may behave bizarrely, for example they may talk to themselves, talk of things which do not make sense or seem unusual. They may get annoyed if others try to reason with them and may not sleep or eat well.

What is mental illness?

All of us face problems in life at some time which can make us feel worried, upset or even angry. For example, when a person has had difficult times at work, they may appear tired, seem angry and irritable. They may even have aches and pains, eat or sleep too little or too much.

These are some mental health difficulties which people can usually overcome and get better. Usually they go away in a few hours or days. Most people get through these times by talking with their families or friends.

However, sometimes these difficulties and behaviours do not get better or seem to get a bit out of hand. People can begin to behave in rather extreme ways, for example not eating, not sleeping or hurting themselves. This change in behaviour may be because the person might have a severe mental illness. At these times they may need help from professionals or a specialist. They may also need some medicines to help.

How do people with a mental illness feel?

It is very difficult to understand or explain how a person with a mental illness feels. The type of illness they have can also influence how they feel. For example, when a person is depressed, it may seem that they are upset with other people, but in reality he or she feels just very unhappy inside without really knowing why.

What causes mental illness?

There is usually no one specific cause for mental illness. A mixture of different things can lead to a person developing a mental illness.

- How a person's body works and functions (their physical health, certain chemicals or changes in their brain).
- Stress or difficulties, for example the break up of an important relationship, losing someone or physical illness.
- Another way of understanding mental illness is to consider it as an imbalance that occurs in the brain. The brain can normally filter out unnecessary information and pay attention to what is needed. Too many worries, thoughts and experiences could cause an overload in the brain. This in turn might lead the mind to feel jumbled up, and the person might experience strange thoughts and ideas which don't fit.

Will I inherit mental illness from my parent or relative?

It is unlikely that mental illness is caused solely by genes or parents passing it on to children. There are no genetic tests for the illness. Remember that even if both your parents have a mental illness, you are still much more likely NOT to have a mental illness than have it. However, some severe mental illnesses are more likely to occur within the same family than others.

Will I get mentally ill from doing drugs/alcohol?

Although it is unlikely that drugs cause permanent mental illness, they can trigger or increase the chance and risk of developing mental health problems. Heavy drug use, including alcohol, could affect your memory permanently. It is unwise to use cannabis regularly or heavily in your teenage years. Research has shown that people who are already at risk of developing mental health problems are more likely to start showing symptoms of mental illness if they use cannabis regularly.

How do I know if someone has a mental illness?

Often people who are mentally ill either don't realise that they are getting ill or don't want people to know about it – so they try their best to manage.

You may realise they have a mental illness if they or someone close (other parent/family/friend) has spoken to you about their illness. You may have noticed they have been to see doctors or gone to hospital without any obvious physical injury or illness. Sometimes you might have noticed they are talking or behaving differently (as described under different types of mental illness).

What do I do if I am worried about my parent or relative's mental health?

If you notice they seem unwell, you could **ask them how they are** and whether they are getting the right help. You may also find it helpful to **speak to your other parent** or close relative – try talking to your dad or grandparents if your mum is unwell.

If there is no other adult (family/friend) around, you may **speak to your GP** (family doctor). Sometimes a professional is already involved in the person's treatment, and you may be able to contact them and let them know your worries. Remember, GPs/professionals may not be able to do anything against the wishes of your parent or relative.

If at any time you feel really frightened by your parent or relative's behaviour (either towards you/others or towards themselves) and you are unable to contact an adult, a doctor or a social worker who can help, you should dial 999. You may feel bad about this but it might be the only way to get the help the person needs.

What can I do if I find things difficult?

You can try a few things.

- Talk to someone whom you trust and who can help. Simply talking to someone you trust, and who you feel understands, can lighten the burden.

- School may be able to help by contacting your parents or setting reminders for special events like trips or plays at school, so you do not miss out.

- Try to get help and support so that you are not on your own taking care of your parent. Sharing the problems can make it easier to work out practical solutions to deal with issues such as how to get to school and back home again, finishing your homework, sorting out meals, etc.

- Try to make sure you do some physical activity, eat healthy food, and allow for fun and leisure time.

- Try to keep yourself occupied by doing your usual activities (homework, meeting friends) as far as possible, even though you may be worried and wish to stay home and be with your parent.

Who else can help me?

You may feel stressed out by your parent's/relative's illness and the behaviour it produces. School nurses or school counsellors can be very helpful in talking all this through with you, and being there if you need to get things off your chest or ask for advice.

You may be able to speak to the professional(s) such as the community mental health nurse who is looking after (treats) your parent. They may be able to answer questions and explain about your parent's illness to you. They may even be able to get you in touch with other young people in similar situations, or organise activities/help for you.

In most local areas there are usually projects and some support available for young people who, just like you, are caring for and worried about a parent/relative with a mental illness. These are usually called 'young carers' projects.

Jessica, 19, talks about her mum who has depression

'I was 12 when my mum started behaving differently. She started ignoring me. She wasn't interested in me ... my food, clothes, chatting – well, anything at all. It seemed to start slowly and I thought she was angry that I had not listened to her about tidying the clothes in my room or something like that. But then, whatever I did she just managed a brief smile, like she would give a stranger. I just felt unloved.

Whatever I did, she wasn't happy. She stopped going out and stayed at home in her room most of the time. When Kim, my 20-year-old sister, came to see us, she tried to talk to her but mum wasn't bothered. Kim spent some time with me, taking me out shopping and cooking a meal. But then she was off. She lived a long way away with her boyfriend and had her college to attend.

Life became an effort for me. I was always late for school, went with my clothes not ironed, and spent my time worrying about my mum in lessons. My teacher noticed this and then I spoke to my learning mentor. One day she came to our home and spoke to my mum. A few days later my mum went to her GP. I'm not sure what happened but then we received an appointment to go to the child and adolescent mental health team and a nurse started visiting us at home. Over the next few months, life seemed back on track.

Looking back, I understand my mum's depression now. But when I was 12, it was different. It was strange ... my mum wasn't the person I knew. I was angry she didn't care about me and upset for not being able to have nice food, clothes or go out with friends.

My teacher had helped to find us the support we needed. My mum still has times when things go downhill, but she gets help early and sees her nurse regularly.' ✪

Recommended reading

Other factsheets in this series:
Coping with stress, Exercise and mental health, When bad things happen, Worries and anxieties

Mental Illness in Your Family, an information booklet from the charity Young Minds. It has a list of where you can get help, as well as more information about various types of mental illness. You can order a paper copy from their website (www.youngminds.org.uk/training_services/publication) or download a free PDF (www.dawsonmarketing.co.uk/youngminds/shop/PDF/B04.pdf).

Minds, Myths and ME, a booklet produced by four British young carers, available from the Royal College of Psychiatrists: www.rcpsych.ac.uk/mentalhealthinfo/youngpeople/caringforyoungcarers.aspx

The Wise Mouse by Virginia Ironside. A storybook explanation of mental illness in parents, for children from 5 to 11 years old. Also available from Young Minds: www.youngminds.org.uk/training_services/publication

When a Parent has a Mental Illness... a 16-minute film which gives demonstrations and explanations of mental illness for children and young people. Produced by Dr Alan Cooklin. It can be viewed or downloaded from the Royal College of Psychiatrists' website: www.rcpsych.ac.uk/mentalhealthinfoforall/youngpeople/caringforaparent.aspx

References

Bailey S, Shooter M. *The Young Mind: An Essential Guide to Mental Health for Parents, Teachers and Young Adults*. Bantam Press, 2009.

Cooklin A. *Being Seen and Heard: The Needs of Children of Parents with Mental Illness* (CD-ROM). RCPsych Publications, 2006. (Multimedia training pack for use of staff involved with parents and their children.)

Persaud R (ed.) *The Mind: A User's Guide*. Bantam Press, 2007.

Useful website

➲ **Young Carers Net**: www.youngcarers.net; online support for young people who care for others from the Princess Royal Trust for Carers.

Notes

....

....

....

....

....

....

....

....

For a catalogue of public education materials or copies of our leaflets contact: Book Sales/Leaflets, The Royal College of Psychiatrists, 17 Belgrave Square, London SW1X 8PG. Email: leaflets@rcpsych.ac.uk, tel: 020 7235 2351 ext. 6146.

Revised by the Royal College of Psychiatrists' Child and Family Public Education Editorial Board. With grateful thanks to Dr Fareeha Amber Sadiq. This leaflet reflects the best possible evidence at the time of writing.

9 Obsessive–compulsive disorder (OCD)
Information for young people

This is one in a series of factsheets for young people, with practical, up-to-date information about mental health problems (emotional, behavioural and psychiatric disorders) that can affect children and young people.

This factsheet describes what obsessive–compulsive disorder is and how it might affect you. It offers practical advice about how to get help.

What are the symptoms?

Obsessions

An obsession is a thought, image or urge that keeps coming into your mind even though you may not want it to. An obsession can be annoying, unpleasant or distressing and you may want it to go away. An example of an obsession is the thought that your hands are dirty even though they are not.

Different people have different obsessions – here are some examples:

- fears about dirt and spreading disease
- worrying about harm happening to you or someone else
- fearing that something 'bad' may happen
- worrying about things being tidy
- worrying about having an illness.

Having an obsession often leads to anxiety or feeling uncomfortable and you may then have the urge to 'put it right'. This is where compulsions come in.

> ### What is obsessive–compulsive disorder (OCD)?
>
> The word 'obsessive' gets used commonly. This can mean different things to different people. Obsessive–compulsive disorder is a type of anxiety disorder. A person with OCD has obsessions and/or compulsions that affect their everyday life, for example going to school on time, finishing homework or being out with friends.

Compulsions

Compulsions are things you feel you need to do usually to control your 'obsessions', even though you may not want to. You might even try to stop doing them, but this might not be possible.

Often, a compulsion means doing something again and again as a 'ritual'. By doing the compulsion, you feel you can prevent or reduce your anxiety about what you fear may happen if you don't do it. For example, turning the light on and off 20 times because you worry something bad may happen if you don't.

Different people have different compulsions. Some examples include:

- washing
- checking
- thinking certain thoughts
- touching
- ordering/arranging things or lining things up
- counting.

People who have these problems often try to avoid any situation that might set off these obsessive thoughts (e.g. not using hands to open doors). When obsessions and compulsions take up a lot of your time, interfere with your life and cause you distress, it may mean you have OCD.

Who does OCD affect?

Obsessive–compulsive disorder is common and can affect people of all ages irrespective of their background (gender, religion, class).

What causes OCD?

We do not know the cause of OCD for certain. However, research suggests that OCD may be due to an imbalance of a brain chemical called serotonin. It is likely that there may be someone in your family who has a similar disorder or have tics (jerky movements).

Sometimes the symptoms seem to start after a specific type of infection (e.g. cough, cold). It can also occur after a difficult time in your life, like having an accident.

How is OCD treated?

There are psychological treatments and medications available to treat OCD. One of the helpful psychological or talking treatments for OCD is **cognitive–behavioural therapy** (CBT) that includes **exposure and response prevention** (ERP). Cognitive–behavioural therapy is a psychological approach that is effective in treating young people with OCD.

People who have OCD often think that by avoiding a certain situation or doing the ritual/compulsion the worry (obsession) will be kept away (or come true). However, this does not help the worry to go away. In the treatment for OCD, the therapist would help you to understand this and also teach you ways to face the worry rather than running away from it. Eventually, this helps to get rid of your obsessions and compulsions.

In ERP the therapist helps you to face the things that you fear and that you have been avoiding. They then help you to stop responding in your usual way (like not letting you wash hands when you worry they are dirty). To help you fight OCD, you will be taught a wide range of skills to manage the anxiety that OCD creates. This helps you to learn strategies to control the OCD rather than it controlling you.

Sometimes the therapist may suggest someone in your family to be involved during the therapy.

When OCD is severe or you struggle with doing the psychological treatment, you may need medication. This is usually given to help along with the CBT. Medication can help you get the most out of the psychological treatment.

How can I get help?

It is important to seek help early and remember that having OCD does not mean you are 'mad' and 'losing control'.

If you are worried about yourself, you should talk to someone you trust, such as your parents or carers, or a teacher. A lot of adults with OCD never got any help for their problems when younger, and now wish they had.

Your GP or school nurse can give you advice and help you get specialist help from the child and adolescent mental health service (CAMHS). They will talk with you in order to understand the difficulties you are experiencing.

It can be hard or embarrassing to discuss the details of your obsessions or compulsions, but giving as much detail as possible will help the therapist or psychiatrist to give you the right treatment. If your life has become severely affected by OCD, you may also need assistance from other professionals, for example teachers, to help you get back to ordinary life at school or college.

Noah, 18, talks about his OCD

'It started without me really noticing it. I got anxious about someone in my family dying – so I began to tap three times when I got worried, for good luck, and that would calm me down. Then I had to do it before I could go to sleep at night – not once but 3 x 3.

When I watched the programme on TV about those germs in hospital it began to get worse. I couldn't tell my mum or dad about it because it sounded so silly. I had to wash my hands all the time because I thought I would pass on an infection and someone would die. It was mainly at home, but then I began to worry that I would catch something at school.

I made my mum wash my school uniform every day. She tried to say no, but I would get so worked up that she would give in. It came to a head when I couldn't get to school on time because I was spending hours in the bathroom in the morning. I had to wash my hair three times as well as going through washing in a set order. If I was interrupted because someone needed the bathroom, I had to start again.

Mum got me some help. I didn't want to be seen as some psycho person, but the doctor was really nice and understood why I was so worked up about everything. That was when I was 14. Now I am 18. It was hard work doing the therapy. It is called CBT. You have to try and work out why you are so anxious and try and control it. Now I am at college and doing a course that I like. I still do some counting, but I can keep it under control.' ✪

Recommended reading

Other factsheets in this series: Coping with stress, Worries and anxieties, When bad things happen, CBT, CAMHS

National Institute for Health and Clinical Excellence, *Treating Obsessive–Compulsive Disorder (OCD) and Body Dysmorphic Disorder (BDD) in Adults, Children and Young People. Understanding NICE Guidance* (2005) – information for people with OCD or BDD, their families and carers, and the public.

The Young Mind: An Essential Guide to Mental Health for Young Adults, Parents and Teachers, edited by Sue Bailey and Mike Shooter (2009) – an accessible, user-friendly handbook produced by the Royal College of Psychiatrists.

References

Fineberg N, Brown A. Pharmaco-therapy for obsessive–compulsive disorder. *Adv Psychiatr Treat* 2011; 17: 419–34.

National Institute for Health and Clinical Excellence. *Core Interventions in the Treatment of Obsessive Compulsive Disorder and Body Dysmorphic Disorder* (CG31). NICE, 2005.

Veale D. Cognitive–behavioural therapy for obsessive–compulsive disorder. *Adv Psychiatr Treat* 2007; 13: 438–46.

Useful websites

➲ **OCD Action**: www.ocdaction.org.uk; national charity for people with OCD.

➲ **OCD Youth Info**: www.ocdyouth.info; a website written by and for young people with OCD, giving information on the disorder and its treatments.

Notes

10 Psychosis
Information for young people

This is one in a series of factsheets for young people, with practical, up-to-date information about mental health problems (emotional, behavioural and psychiatric disorders) that can affect children and young people.

This factsheet describes psychosis, and how and why it might affect you. It also offers some practical advice about how to get help.

How do I know if I have psychosis?

When you have psychosis, you will often have very unusual and sometimes unpleasant thoughts and experiences. They may appear suddenly making you feel really frightened. They can also creep in so gradually that others, for instance your close family and friends, notice you are behaving strangely before you know it yourself.

You may experience one or more of the symptoms described below.

- **Unusual beliefs called 'delusions'** These are very strong beliefs which are obviously untrue to others, but not to you. For example, when you are ill, you may think that there is a plot to harm you or that you are being spied on by the TV or being taken over by aliens. Sometimes you may feel you have special powers.

- **Thought disorder** This is when you cannot think straight. Your ideas may seem jumbled, but it is more than being muddled or confused. Other people will find it very difficult to follow what you say.

- **Unusual experiences called 'hallucinations'** These are when you can see, hear, smell or feel something that isn't really there. The most common hallucination that people have is hearing voices. Hallucinations are very real to the person having them. This can be very frightening and can make you believe that you are being watched or picked on.

Having these strange thoughts and experiences can affect you at school, at home or when you are with friends. You may find it difficult to concentrate and enjoy your usual activities. They can even affect your sleep and appetite.

What is psychosis?

Young people often worry that they may be 'going mad' when they are feeling stressed, confused or very upset. In fact, worries like this are rarely a sign of mental illness. 'Psychosis' is when your thoughts are so disturbed that you lose touch with reality. This can be severe and distressing.

How common is it?

Psychosis affects people of all ages, but is rare before you reach the older teenage years.

What causes psychosis?

When you have a psychotic episode, it can be a sign of another underlying illness. You can have a psychotic episode after a stressful event such as losing a close friend or relative. It can also be the result of a physical illness (e.g. a severe infection), the use of illegal drugs (e.g. cannabis) or a severe mental illness (e.g. schizophrenia or bipolar disorder).

Sometimes, especially the first time you experience the illness, it is difficult to know what has caused it.

Luke, 16, talks about psychosis

'I was about 14 when it happened. I had a good family, did well at school and had a group of good friends. Life had been good to me, although my mum said I could not handle stress. I would be a bag of nerves before exams, was scared of failing and could not face it if someone was unwell.

Uncle Rob's death a year back in an accident was just too much. I knew I would feel upset for a long time. But then I didn't feel upset. It was strange. I thought people were doing strange things to me like controlling me through radio signals. I felt I had lost control of myself and even felt my body was changing in a strange sort of way ... not just the puberty. And then I could not face school, I was swearing, felt muddled in my head. My learning mentor got worried and spoke to my mum, who had noticed my strange behaviour. I couldn't sleep and couldn't be bothered about going out. I didn't like the idea of seeing a psychiatrist and I thought they would judge me. But it was very different. The psychiatrist seemed to know and understand how I felt, what I thought. I felt relieved. She even said I was not going to be locked away in a hospital. It was just an illness for which I needed to take medication for a few months or a year. She then introduced me to a worker from an early intervention psychosis team. She explained to me and my family all about psychosis, what we could do to keep me well. She was there when I felt I was losing it before my exams.

It's nearly 2 years now. I am like any other 16-year-old, going to school, meeting with friends, etcetera. I take my meds and stay away from drugs and alcohol.' ✪

How do I get help?

It is important that you seek help early. The earlier you are treated for psychosis, the quicker you can get back to your normal life.

First, you could talk to your family, school nurse or GP. They may get you specialist help from a child and adolescent mental health service (CAMHS) team or an early intervention team or service, a specialist team for young people with psychosis.

With psychosis, you often don't realise that you are unwell, but people around you may notice it first. If you become very unwell, you may need to spend some time in hospital until you get better and the illness is under control or goes away completely.

What is the treatment for psychosis?

- Medication

  Medications called 'antipsychotics' are an important part of treatment. They may need to be taken for a long time to stay well. As with medication of any kind, there can be side-effects. The doctor you see will be able to advise you on these and what can be done to help.

  If the psychosis is related to drug use or an underlying physical illness, you may need specific help and treatment to manage this.

- Support

  Other forms of treatment are also important. You and your family will need help to understand more about your illness, how to manage it, and how to help prevent it coming back. You may need support to rebuild your confidence to continue with school, college or work.

- Talking treatments

  Treatments such as cognitive–behavioural therapy can be helpful as well, but need to be undertaken in addition to medication.

What will happen in the future?

Most young people with early help and treatment recover from their psychotic episode. If the illness is due to an underlying physical illness or the use of drugs, you might avoid having another episode by taking the right treatment and avoiding taking drugs.

It is often difficult to know what the long-term effects of a psychotic episode will be and a definite diagnosis may not be possible straight away.

Is there anything else I should do?

It is important to continue with any treatment advised by your doctor and keep a balanced, healthy lifestyle.

Talking to others when you feel stressed can help in identifying problems early and getting the right treatment.

Recommended reading

Other factsheets in this series:
Coping with stress, CBT, CAMHS

Changing Minds. Mental Health: What it is, What to do, Where to go? This is a CD produced by the Royal College of Psychiatrists for 13- to 17-year-olds. It talks about addiction, stress, eating disorders, depression, schizophrenia and self-harm.

The Young Mind: An Essential Guide to Mental Health for Young Adults, Parents and Teachers, edited by Sue Bailey and Mike Shooter (2009) – an accessible, user-friendly handbook produced by the Royal College of Psychiatrists.

References.

National Institute for Health and Clinical Excellence. *Core Interventions in the Treatment and Management of Schizophrenia in Primary and Secondary Care (Update)* (CG82). NICE, 2009.

Rutter M, Bishop D, Pine D, et al (eds) *Rutter's Child and Adolescent Psychiatry* (5th edn). Wiley–Blackwell, 2008

Useful websites

➲ **Talk to Frank**: www.talktofrank.com; helps you find out everything you might want to know about drugs (and some stuff you don't). Helpline: 0800 776600.

➲ **Rethink Mental Illness**: www.rethink.org; offers help to people with severe mental illness (not only psychosis) and their carers.

➲ **Young Minds**: www.youngminds.org.uk; a charity committed to improving the emotional well-being and mental health of children and young people.

Notes

....

....

....

....

....

....

....

....

....

....

For a catalogue of public education materials or copies of our leaflets contact: Book Sales/Leaflets, The Royal College of Psychiatrists, 17 Belgrave Square, London SW1X 8PG. Email: leaflets@rcpsych.ac.uk, tel: 020 7235 2351 ext. 6146.

Revised by the Royal College of Psychiatrists' Child and Family Public Education Editorial Board. We are grateful to the Very Important Kids (VIKs) from Young Minds for commenting on this factsheet and to Dr Vasu Balaguru for updating it. This leaflet reflects the best possible evidence at the time of writing.

11 Schizophrenia
Information for young people

This is one in a series of factsheets for young people, with practical, up-to-date information about mental health problems (emotional, behavioural and psychiatric disorders) that can affect children and young people.

This factsheet describes what schizophrenia is and how and why it might affect you. It also offers some practical advice about how to get help.

What is schizophrenia?

Schizophrenia is a serious illness affecting thoughts, feelings and behaviour. It is a type of psychosis. A lot of people wrongly refer to schizophrenia as having a 'split personality' like Dr Jekyll and Mr Hyde.

How common is it?

Schizophrenia rarely occurs before puberty and usually begins in the late teenage years. About 1 in 100 people will have schizophrenia over their lifetime.

How do I know if I have schizophrenia?

When a person has schizophrenia, they may have the difficulties described below as 'positive' or 'negative' symptoms. Some of the symptoms may seem to start suddenly, whereas others may creep in more gradually. You may have some or most of the following. Usually people have a few or most symptoms for some time (at least months) before they are diagnosed with schizophrenia.

Positive symptoms

This does not mean they are 'good' symptoms. They mean unusual thoughts or experiences as described below. They may feel really distressing. They can feel totally real to you and it may seem to you that other people don't understand or aren't taking you seriously.

- Unusual beliefs or **delusions**: these are beliefs which seem obviously untrue to others, but not to you. For example, when you are ill, you might strongly believe that there is a plot to harm you, you are being spied on through the TV or being taken over by aliens. These beliefs can obviously make you feel afraid or strange.

- **Muddled thinking** or **thought disorder** is when it is difficult to think straight. Sometimes it may feel that others do not understand what you are trying to say. Your ideas may feel jumbled up, but it is more than being muddled or confused.

- Unusual experiences called **hallucinations** are when you see, hear, smell or feel something that isn't really there, although you are convinced that it is. 'Hearing voices' is one of the most common hallucinations. This can be very frightening. It can make you believe that you are being 'watched' or 'picked on'. Your friends or family may say that you are acting strangely. They may say that they hear you talking or laughing to yourself. Sometimes this is the only symptom you experience which makes it unlikely to be schizophrenia.

Negative symptoms

This does not mean they are 'bad' symptoms, just that they are about 'not doing' something. You may feel tired, not interested and not want to do normal things such as:

- go to school
- play sports
- see friends
- get washed and dressed
- do hobbies you used to enjoy.

> **Justin, 19, talks about his illness**
>
> 'I was in year 10 with big dreams about my future. I worked hard, studying, wanting to do my best. Over time I felt I had special skills and powers. I could work like a genius, I was keen to make a discovery, I was sure that I was on my way to becoming the youngest Nobel prizewinner. I couldn't be bothered by my friends who were just ordinary people. I started hearing special messages through the computer giving me a new formula for my discovery. I had to keep this a secret, be sure not even my family knew all the work I was doing. I was sure there were spies who wished to get the formula and to make money out of it.
>
> My mother thought I was crazy. She wanted me to go to college but I had better plans. Then one day she said I had to see my doctor. I was really angry, but in another way she was right. I looked at myself in the mirror, it was not me and it felt strange.
>
> I met a doctor, a shrink. I thought they were all against me, didn't understand me. I refused to see them, but only agreed for my family's sake. There was one part of me which felt like I was in a dream, something was not right.
>
> Slowly it started unfolding … all those thoughts were crazy. It was never me … I agreed to take some medication at least to help me sleep and not feel scared at night thinking the spies wanted me or my work. A few weeks later my head was clearer. I felt really ashamed and was unsure what I would do in future. I had schizophrenia. I thought I would end it all. I wanted to run away.
>
> The psychiatrist and a worker from the early intervention team were very patient. They explained the illness to me. I even spoke to people with similar experiences as me. I am in college now, I have a girlfriend and I am living in a flat with staff who help me. It has been a long, difficult journey, but it's not as bad as I thought. I feel happy my mum got me the right help and was there for me all the way.' ✪

Other symptoms

- You may become frustrated and angry, especially towards your friends or family.
- Some people try to smoke or drink alcohol to feel better, but this tends to make things worse.

You may find the symptoms so distressing that you feel like harming yourself.

What causes schizophrenia?

This is still not fully understood. There are a number of reasons that can make a person more likely to develop schizophrenia or a similar psychotic illness.

- There may be chemical imbalances in the brain.
- Having a parent or close relative suffering from schizophrenia can increase the chance of developing a similar illness.
- Stress or extreme life events (like someone close dying).
- Using drugs like cannabis, LSD, ecstasy and speed (amphetamine).

What is the treatment for schizophrenia?

- Medications called **'antipsychotics'** are an important part of treatment and often need to be taken for a long time to stay well. As with medication of any kind, there may be side-effects. The doctor will be able to advise you on what they are and what can be done to help.

  If you are taking drugs like cannabis, it is very important that you stop.
- Other forms of treatment are also important. Both you and your family will need help to understand the condition, to cope successfully and to prevent the illness coming back. **Support** is often needed to rebuild your confidence to continue with school, college or work.
- You may be referred to a specialist **early intervention service** (EIS) if available locally. This is a team of specialists who help young people with psychosis. You also may at some point need treatment in hospital or in a specialist in-patient service.
- **Talking treatments** can be helpful, but are usually offered in addition to medication.

What will happen in the future?

Schizophrenia is a chronic illness, which means that even if you get better, it might come back later on. This can happen if you stop taking your medication too soon, so it is really important to follow the advice given to you by your doctor.

Your child and adolescent mental health service (CAMHS) or early intervention team will also help you and your family identify ways to help prevent the illness coming back (e.g. following a healthy lifestyle, learning to cope with stress).

Most young people will recover from their illness with the right help and treatment. Earlier treatment leads to better recovery and increases the chances of finishing school or college, getting a job and getting on with life.

How do I get help?

- It is important to speak to someone you trust and who possibly knows you well, such as your GP or teacher. They may not believe or agree with your strange beliefs or experiences, but they can still help you by listening and getting the right help for you.

- It is also possible that your family or teachers will first seek help for you as you may not notice there is a problem, and find it difficult to accept that there is something wrong.

- Often you will be asked to get specialist help. A CAMHS member or psychiatrist from CAMHS may need to see you to understand and assess your difficulties before treating the illness.

Recommended reading

Other factsheets in this series: Cannabis and mental health, Psychosis, Worries and anxieties, CAMHS

The Young Mind: An Essential Guide to Mental Health for Young Adults, Parents and Teachers, edited by Sue Bailey and Mike Shooter (2009) – an accessible, user-friendly handbook produced by the Royal College of Psychiatrists.

References

National Institute for Health and Clinical Excellence. *Core Interventions in the Treatment and Management of Schizophrenia in Primary and Secondary Care (Update)* (CG82). NICE, 2009.

Rutter M, Bishop D, Pine D, et al (eds). *Rutter's Child and Adolescent Psychiatry* (5th edn). Wiley–Blackwell, 2008.

Useful websites

- ⊃ **Mind**: www.mind.org.uk; a national mental health charity for England and Wales.

- ⊃ **Sane**: www.sane.org.uk; provides practical help to improve quality of life for people affected by mental illness

- ⊃ **Young Minds**: www.youngminds.org.uk; a charity committed to improving the emotional well-being and mental health of children and young people.

Notes

For a catalogue of public education materials or copies of our leaflets contact: Book Sales/Leaflets, The Royal College of Psychiatrists, 17 Belgrave Square, London SW1X 8PG. Email: leaflets@rcpsych.ac.uk, tel: 020 7235 2351 ext. 6146.

Revised by the Royal College of Psychiatrists' Child and Family Public Education Editorial Board. We are grateful to the Very Important Kids (VIKs) from Young Minds for commenting on this factsheet and to Dr Vasu Balaguru for updating it. This leaflet reflects the best possible evidence at the time of writing.

12 When bad things happen – overcoming adversity and developing resilience
Information for young people

This is one in a series of factsheets for young people, with practical, up-to-date information about mental health problems (emotional, behavioural and psychiatric disorders) that can affect children and young people.

This factsheet explains what difficulties you can face and what to do when bad things happen.

What does it mean to have resilience?

Bad things happen to everyone. These experiences may be very difficult, yet some children show a remarkable ability to manage and cope. We call these children 'resilient'. Some children can be more resilient than others which may explain why children within the same family may react differently to a traumatic event, such as a death in the family. This leaflet is about building resilience and finding ways to cope better with difficult situations.

When bad things happen, you may feel sad and worried, angry and stressed. Life can become tough sometimes, so learning how to cope is an important skill we need to have. If life was always perfect then we would never develop coping skills or learn what makes us feel better. So dealing with difficulties can help us learn how to cope with problems when they crop up, as we know what works for us.

Having a friend to talk to, having an interest which distracts us from our worries, chilling out by listening to music or surfing the net can all be ways of coping.

What do you do when things are tough?

There are some things specific to you that will affect how you manage situations such as those described in the box on the right. These are not things you can change, but they may explain why you might find your situation more difficult than your brother or sister does. For example, you may have an illness yourself, such as asthma or diabetes, which is an added stress; or you may tend to be a 'worrier' rather than someone who is more 'easy going'. Neither is better overall, but being more of a worrier may mean you feel more affected by things that happen in your life.

How can I make things easier for myself?

Things that make life difficult are often completely out of your control. But there are things you can do to make them have less of an effect on you. This doesn't mean managing things on your own, but asking for help, sometimes even outside your family. You could start by confiding in someone you trust. If that doesn't work, you could try other things.

- Spend more time doing something you enjoy and are good at. This may be something you do at school, for example, your favourite subject, or it may be a sport such as football, swimming or dancing, or another activity like music.

- Use a grown-up outside the close family, such as a teacher, a youth worker, a grandparent or a social worker for support. If you can't think of anyone, your school or local council services may provide a mentor.

What are 'bad' things?

There are lots of things that can make life tough, often things that are not in your control. Usually, the difficulty will involve your family, your friends, your neighbourhood or your school, as these are the people and places that have the most effect on you as you grow older.

Below is a list of the sorts of problems we are talking about:

- having an ill parent
- parents who fight and argue a lot
- losing a parent
- parents divorcing
- parents who drink a lot of alcohol or take street drugs
- parent/friend who is in trouble with the police
- friends who take street drugs
- your family trying to manage without enough money
- living in an area where you don't feel safe, or see or experience violence
- living away from your parents, e.g. in foster care or a children's home
- being bullied
- being physically or sexually abused.

Several of these problems can happen together which makes it more difficult to cope.

Jamie, 12, talks about his brother's illness

'Everything changed in my life when Billy got sick. We were fine, me, Mum, Billy. Then next thing, he's in hospital and Mum's all over the place. He got some sort of cancer. He was only 8.

Suddenly, I had to sort everything out at home. Mum was hardly ever around early on, and even when she was, she wasn't really. She was really worried. She'd cry a lot too. I did loads more at home to try to help. Washing, buying food and stuff. But it was tough. I was worried too.

At school, they knew something was up. I was late a lot and didn't get my work done on time. I didn't get to football practice. My head of year called me in for a chat. He was really helpful. I told him what was going on with Billy. He knew Dad wasn't around anymore and asked if anyone else could help out a bit. I told him that after Nan died, we didn't really have anyone else. So he saw I had a lot on my plate.

He phoned Mum. He wasn't interfering, just trying to help. He said they were missing me at football and told her how good I was. Then he said it'd be good for me to go to homework club more, so I could get my work done and she could stay at the hospital with Billy for longer.

They were only little things when you think about it, but they really helped. I could be myself again, playing football, even if it was just for a few hours a week. I wasn't as behind with my work either. And my head of year kept an eye on me. I went to see him if I was having a rough day. It was good he knew about Billy; I didn't have to keep explaining.

Billy's home now. He's not better yet, but he's getting there. And he's so brave about it all, he makes me feel stronger just being with him.' ✪

Encourage your family to keep doing the things that make you have a happy time together, even if you are all struggling through a difficult situation. This will help you to feel closer and warmer towards each other.

• Think about joining an after-school activity club in your neighbourhood. This will let you have fun safely, and may give you time away from stress at home or with friends. You may also make different friends who may be more supportive.

What if this isn't enough?

If you try these ways of helping yourself and you still do not feel any better, or your situation does not improve, it may be that it is just too much for you to manage on your own. It could be that your difficulties are so stressful that they have triggered an illness like depression or anxiety.

Who can I turn to for help?

Coping with the problems we have mentioned is not easy. It is in no way a sign of weakness if you feel you cannot manage on your own; it is more a sign of strength that you know when to ask for help.

The best people to ask for help will be other adults you know. This could mean:

• your teacher
• your head of year
• your school nurse
• a school counsellor or youth worker
• a family member
• a family friend.

The adult you confide in will think through your situation with you, and will think about whether other people might be able to help. This might mean help for you, help for your parents, or for the whole family. The people who may become involved include:

• your GP or practice nurse
• a local counselling service
• your local child and adolescent mental health service (CAMHS), who are a team of professionals specially trained to work with young people
• a family social worker.

These people work in different ways to each other, but all will aim to support you and improve the situation for you and your family.

Recommended reading

Other factsheets in this series:
Coping with stress, Depression,
Worries and anxieties, CAMHS

*The Young Mind: An Essential
Guide to Mental Health for
Young Adults, Parents and
Teachers*, edited by Sue Bailey
and Mike Shooter (2009) –
an accessible, user-friendly
handbook produced by the
Royal College of Psychiatrists.

References

Goodman R, Scott S. *Child
Psychiatry* (2nd edn). Wiley-
Blackwell, 2005.

Rutter M, Bishop D, Pine D, et
al (eds) *Rutter's Child and
Adolescent Psychiatry* (5th edn).
Wiley–Blackwell, 2008.

Useful websites

- ➲ **Childline**: www.childline.org.uk; provides a 24-hour free and confidential telephone, email and chat service for children and young people. Helpline: 0800 1111.
- ➲ **Samaritans**: www.samaritans.org; offers confidential, 24-hour emotional support to anyone in a crisis. UK helpline: 08457 909090, Irish helpline: 1850 609090, email: jo@samaritans.org.
- ➲ **Teenage Health Freak**: www.teenagehealthfreak.org; accurate and reliable health information for teenagers.

Notes

_____

_____

_____

_____

_____

_____

_____

_____

13 Worries about weight and eating problems
Information for young people

This is one in a series of factsheets for young people, with practical, up-to-date information about mental health problems (emotional, behavioural and psychiatric disorders) that can affect children and young people.

This factsheet looks at some of the reasons why young people worry about their weight. It offers advice about how to maintain a normal and healthy weight and not let these worries get out of control.

How do I stay healthy and have a normal weight?

Our bodies need a healthy diet which should include all the things you need to develop normally – proteins, carbohydrates, fats, minerals and vitamins. Cutting out things you might see as fattening, such as carbohydrates or fats, can stop your body from developing normally.

There are some simple rules that can help you to keep a healthy weight. They sound quite easy, but might be more difficult to put into practice. You can ask your family and friends to help you to stick to these rules. It might even help them to be a bit healthier!

- Eat regular meals – breakfast, lunch and dinner. Include carbohydrate foods such as bread, potatoes, rice or pasta with every meal.
- Try to eat at the same times each day. Long gaps between meals can make you so hungry that you eventually eat far more than you need to.
- Get enough sleep.
- Avoid sugary or high-fat foods and junk foods. If you have a lunch of crisps, chocolate and a soft drink, it doesn't feel as if you're eating much, but it will pile on the pounds. A sandwich, fruit and milk or juice will fill you up, but you are much less likely to put on weight – and it's better for your skin.
- Take regular exercise. Cycling, walking or swimming are all good ways of staying fit without going over the top.
- Try not to pay too much attention to other people who skip meals or talk about their weight.

If you follow these suggestions, you will find it easier to control your weight, and you won't find yourself wanting sweet foods all the time.

What about 'miracle cures' for losing weight – do they work?

There seems to be a new one of these almost every week. Sadly, they often do more harm than good.

- Crash diets don't help you to keep your weight down. In fact, they might make you put on weight after a while. At worst, they can be dangerous to your health.
- Exercise helps, but it's got to be regular and increased gradually. Too much exercise, or too much too soon, can damage your body.
- Laxatives might help you feel less guilty and bloated. Unfortunately, they don't reduce weight and can upset your body chemistry.
- 'Slimming pills' can't make you thinner. They might make you feel a bit less hungry, but unfortunately, they can also harm your health.

Why do people worry about weight?

Most of us, at some time in our lives, feel unhappy about the way we look and try to change it. Being smaller, shorter or less well-developed than friends or brothers and sisters can make us feel anxious and lacking in confidence. So can being teased about your size and weight. Many of us have an idea of the size and shape we would like to be.

Our ideas about what looks good are strongly influenced by fashion and friends. You might compare yourself with the pictures in magazines. The models in these magazines are often unhealthily thin. You may then worry that you are fat, even if your weight is normal for your age and height.

There are a variety of sizes and shapes that are within the normal, healthy range. If you are interested, there are tables showing normal height and weight. Ask your school nurse, GP or library. Your weight, like your height and looks, depends a lot on your build, your genes and your diet.

What causes problems with eating?

Problems or pressures at school, with friends or at home are common causes of problems with eating. Your appetite can be affected by stress, pressure, worry or tiredness.

Some people turn to food for comfort. This can lead to eating more than we need and can make us put on weight. It's easy to start worrying about getting fat and we find ourselves eating even more to comfort ourselves. It becomes a vicious circle. 'Comfort foods' often contain a lot of fat or sugar – sweets, biscuits, chocolate, cakes and pastries. It can be helpful to keep a diary of what you eat to make sure that you don't slip into this.

If you are unhappy or stressed, it can be easy to focus on your weight and eating habits instead of the things that are bothering you. If this goes on for long enough, you might develop an eating disorder.

What are the different types of eating disorder?

The most common eating disorder is becoming overweight (obesity). Other eating disorders are less common. Anorexia nervosa and bulimia nervosa occur most often among girls, but can happen in boys too.

If worries have altered your appetite or weight, it will help to talk to someone.

How do I know if I have an eating disorder?

When you have an eating disorder you may notice some of the signs listed below.

If you have anorexia

- You may be exercising a lot more than usual to lose weight
- You feel afraid of putting on weight
- You don't feel good about yourself and the way you look
- If you are female, your periods may be irregular or may have stopped
- You may have noticed changes in your physical health
- You will feel you are fat and will avoid eating, even though you aren't actually overweight
- You feel guilty when you eat
- You avoid food, lose a lot of weight and become extremely thin.

Annabelle, 16

'I'm 16 now, but I think I started having a problem when I was 12. I became very worried about my weight and my body. I had put on a bit of weight and was very upset when a boy in my class called me fat. I remember feeling that even if I was doing very well in school, things weren't quite right and I wasn't quite good enough.

Gradually I ate less, lost masses of weight, but still believed that I was fat. Sometimes I "felt" fat and this made me feel very down. I stopped seeing most of my friends, and spent more and more time thinking about food and my body.

I was always checking the shape of my stomach and bottom – 20 or 30 times a day, looking at them in great detail. I felt very cold at times, and found it harder and harder to find the energy to do things as I was eating less and less.

I also weighed myself at least 5 times a day, and if my weight had not gone down, I checked my stomach, and tried dieting even more. Sometimes I binged on cakes and chocolate. I felt very guilty afterwards and would usually be sick so that I could get rid of the food and lose some weight. It felt as if I was going round and round in circles, with no means of escape.

One of my teachers noticed that I wasn't eating lunch and that I had become thin (or at least she thought I had). She spoke to my parents and I was taken to a clinic. At first I didn't want to know and I didn't want to be helped. However, I started a treatment called cognitive–behavioural therapy. I learnt to look at the links between my thoughts, feelings and behaviour, but more importantly, I learnt that I could eat regularly, without putting on weight.

Gradually, I put on some weight and worked on my checking and weighing behaviour. It wasn't easy to get better. I slowly started to eat the foods that I used to avoid. Sometimes I still find myself thinking the way I used to, but now I know that this is only one way of thinking, one way of being, and most of the time choose not to do this.

I love going out clubbing with my friends now and I don't argue quite so much with my parents, well at least not about food anyway.' ✪

Janet, 18

'Two years ago it was my "best friend" and now it's my "enemy"! It no longer controls me or my family and together we've pushed it away. I couldn't have done it alone. I wouldn't have made it to the unit if it wasn't for my mum and the school nurse who convinced me to see a professional team…that took them 6 months!…I was really pig-headed! I am talking about anorexia.

It started when I was 15 and my friends and I tried the "South Beach" diet…most of them dropped out but I stuck with it…I've always been competitive.

At home there was so much pressure to get "A" grades; at last, there was a different focus. I became obsessed with counting calories and even kept a food diary. I lost more weight but still felt huge and "ugly" and wanted to lose more…My friends tried to stop me and said they were worried, but I didn't care.

Slowly, I stopped going out with them, preferring to stay in and do my sit-up regime. I thought about taking slimming pills but was too scared so I bought laxatives instead. I felt so driven to lose weight; the thought of putting on an ounce scared me to death. I remember feeling weepy and very tired. At its worst, my fingers and toes went blue!

Then, I agreed to see the child and family mental health service where I met a team of professionals including a nurse, psychiatrist, psychologist and family therapist. They offered me individual therapy every week, to work through things and have my physical health monitored too. The family therapist was also able to offer us time as a family to work things out. This felt like the most important bit for a long time, especially for Dad who found it hard to understand anorexia. It was tough and sometimes we felt like throwing the towel in, but the team supported us and we felt safe. Even now some days are hard, but we got through it.' ✪

Strangely, the thinner you get, the fatter you feel! We don't fully understand why this happens, but it makes the eating disorder harder to overcome.

People with anorexia usually remain very active – and say they are well – even though they become so thin that they avoid undressing in front of others or wear loose clothes to hide their size.

Anorexia nervosa can be dangerous if it gets out of control. If you are a girl and your periods have stopped, this is a warning sign which means you need help right away (this won't happen if you are on the pill – so if you are, don't wait for this before you seek help)!

If you don't eat much, you can feel like you are starving! You may then find yourself bingeing – eating lots of food very quickly. Bingeing also happens in an eating disorder known as bulimia.

If you have bulimia

- You avoid foods such as chocolates, cakes or biscuits, except when you binge.
- You feel fat, guilty and ashamed when you binge.
- You try to get rid of the food by being sick or using laxatives. It usually doesn't make much difference to your weight, but can damage your health and take up a lot of time and energy.

Some people have both anorexic and bulimic symptoms.

What are the consequences of having an eating disorder?

Having an eating disorder can be crippling. It can affect your concentration, education or work as well as social life like going out with friends; all of this has an impact on your emotional and mental health. An eating disorder can also cause severe and serious physical health problems, both in the short and long term.

If you are worried about your weight or feel you might have an eating disorder, you should get some help.

How do I get help?

Talk to:
- a member of the family
- a teacher or school nurse
- a counsellor or social worker
- your GP
- a Beat professional (www.b-eat.co.uk).

Your GP or practice nurse is the best person for basic information and advice on diet and weight. If you need more specialist help, they can refer you to a specialist or suggest that you see a professional at your local child and adolescent mental health service (CAMHS). This is a team of specialists including child and adolescent psychiatrists, psychologists, social workers, psychotherapists and specialist nurses. They can help you to regain control of your eating and your weight. Most young people do get better with help.

Recommended reading

Other factsheets in this series: CAMHS, CBT

Changing Minds. Mental Health: What it is, What to do, Where to go? This is a CD produced by the Royal College of Psychiatrists for 13- to 17-year-olds. It talks about addiction, stress, eating disorders, depression, schizophrenia and self-harm.

The Young Mind: An Essential Guide to Mental Health for Young Adults, Parents and Teachers, edited by Sue Bailey and Mike Shooter (2009) – an accessible, user-friendly handbook produced by the Royal College of Psychiatrists.

References

National Institute for Health and Clinical Excellence. *Eating Disorders: Core Interventions in the Treatment and Management of Anorexia Nervosa, Bulimia Nervosa and Related Eating Disorders.* NICE, 2004.

Rutter M, Bishop D, Pine D, et al (eds) *Rutter's Child and Adolescent Psychiatry* (5th edn). Wiley–Blackwell, 2008.

Useful websites

- **B-eat (beating eating disorders)**: www.b-eat.co.uk; helplines, online support and a network of UK-wide self-help groups to assist adults and young people in the UK in beating their eating disorders. Helpline for young people: 0845 634 7650.

- **Young Minds**: www.youngminds.org.uk; information for young people about mental health and emotional well-being.

Notes

....

....

....

....

....

....

....

....

....

14 Worries and anxieties
Information for young people

This is one in a series of factsheets for young people, with practical, up-to-date information about mental health problems (emotional, behavioural and psychiatric disorders) that can affect children and young people.

This factsheet describes the different types of anxieties that children and young people might feel and some of the reasons for this. It also offers practical advice on how to deal with worries and anxieties.

How common is it?

Anxiety is one of the common mental health problems. Nearly 300 000 young people in Britain have an anxiety disorder. So you are not alone. Lots of people, however, suffer in silence. It is important to recognise your problems and seek help, especially when anxiety starts affecting your everyday life.

What does anxiety feel like?

When we feel we are in danger, our brains tell our bodies to get ready to run away quickly. This means that if you have anxiety you may feel this in your mind, as well as physically in your body.

Some of the most common symptoms of anxiety are listed below.

> ### What is anxiety?
>
> We all get frightened or worried from time to time. Fear can be a good thing as it keeps us from getting too close to danger. Sometimes, we can feel frightened or worry about things too much and this can get in the way of enjoying life. This sort of fear or worry is called anxiety.

In your body you may feel:
- sick
- shaky/dizzy
- your heart racing
- short of breath
- 'butterflies' in the stomach.

In your mind you may:
- feel upset
- feel worried
- feel irritable
- feel unable to relax
- have difficulty in concentrating.

What different types of anxiety can I experience?

Anxieties are grouped based on what the fear or worry is about. Grouping is also helpful in understanding your difficulties and treating them.

Fears and phobias

You might remember being scared of the dark or insects when you were little. This is normal and as we get older, we usually grow out of these fears or are able to manage them without worrying too much about it. Sometimes fears about particular things (e.g. needles, animals) or places (e.g. darkness, heights) can be really strong and don't go away. They stop you from doing normal things and interfere or take over your life. These fears are called phobias. You may need extra help to cope with a phobia.

General anxiety

Some people feel anxious most of the time for no obvious reason. When it is really bad, it can stop you concentrating at school or having fun with friends and family. Sometimes feeling anxious and sad can go together. You may need help to be able to feel and cope better.

Separation anxiety

Separation anxiety is feeling worried or anxious when you are away from your parents/family/guardians. It is normal for very young children to feel scared and worried when they are not with the people who normally look after them. If it is still a problem when you are older or a teenager, this can make it difficult to go to school or go out with friends. If this happens it is best to get help.

Social anxiety

In simple terms this is really bad shyness. You may be comfortable with people you know well, but find it very worrying to be with new people, in new places or social occasions like parties. Speaking up in class or assembly can be extremely difficult for you, as you are worried about making mistakes or what others think of you. This means you may tend to avoid situations which involve other people. When this happens, it is important to seek help.

Panic disorder

A panic attack is an extreme episode of anxiety that seems to occur for no reason. It may feel as if your mind has gone totally out of control. Panic attacks have a start and a finish; they are not continuous, although you might worry about when the next one will happen. During an attack, you can have physical feelings of anxiety along with frightening thoughts, like thinking you are going to die or 'go mad'. It is rare for younger children to have panic attacks on their own, without another form of anxiety such as those mentioned earlier. This becomes more common in teenagers. When the fear of having an attack or having attacks frequently stops you from doing your daily routine or enjoying life, this is called panic disorder.

Other anxieties

Some children and young people may have other types of anxiety, such as post-traumatic stress disorder or obsessive–compulsive disorder.

What causes these worries and anxieties?

We do not really know what causes this illness. However, sometimes you may find that the problems started after upsetting or frightening experiences in your life (e.g. being bullied at school, having an illness, losing someone you love, your parents separating). You may be able to manage one thing, but when lots of things happen at once, like parents separating, moving house and changing school, it can become much more difficult.

Anxiety tends to run in families, so if someone in your family is known to worry a lot, you may be more likely to worry as well. Some of this will be passed on in the genes, but you may also 'learn' anxious behaviour from being around anxious people. If your family or friends are anxious or harsh, it can make your anxiety worse. In this case it may help to talk to them about it.

Will I grow out of it?

Some people may grow out of anxiety, but a few may still experience it when they grow up. The good news is that anxiety is treatable.

What can I do?

There is a lot you can do with the help of family and good friends to make you feel better.

- Try to give yourself more time to get used to any changes that happen at home or at school, as change can be more difficult when you worry a lot.

Neela's story, 15

'I don't know about you, but I have always been a worrier, like my grandmother. Every year, we would plan our family trip to India and it would start…worrying about the plane journey…worrying about falling ill,…and just before take-off I would get those horrible "butterflies", sweaty hands and the feeling that I couldn't breathe. Sometimes I would feel my heart beating and I thought I was dying or going "crazy".

Last year, before my exams, my worrying got really bad. The pressure in secondary school has been high, and everyone in my family has always done well and gone on to university, so I knew I had to study extra hard. It got so bad that I couldn't concentrate. I felt shaky and nervous at school and even started to cry most days. I wasn't sleeping well because I was so nervous and was too embarrassed to tell my mum and dad.

I ended up pouring my heart out to the school nurse which was the best thing I ever did. She got in touch with my mum, and after seeing the GP, I went to see a team of specialists at the hospital.

Don't worry…I didn't want to be the "girl who sees the shrink" either but it's not like that. The team can have all sorts of people like doctors, nurses, psychologists and social workers. They reassured me and helped me and my family to see that my symptoms were real (just like when you have asthma). I went on to have a talking therapy called CBT. This involves a number of weekly sessions with the therapist. I didn't even need to take medication. Although I will always be a worrier, I feel so much better, and I'm even looking forward to this year's India trip!' ✪

- Check if you might be picking up on someone else's worry, rather than it being your own.
- Get support from good friends and family; you might also want to talk to someone outside the family, such as a teacher or mentor.

If this isn't enough, you might need more specialist help. Speak to your GP or school nurse, who may send you to see someone from the local child and adolescent mental health service (CAMHS).

How is anxiety treated?

The type of specialist help offered to you will depend on what is causing the anxiety. Usually it will be a form of **talking therapy**, such as cognitive–behavioural therapy (CBT). Cognitive–behavioural therapy can help you understand and deal with the causes of your anxiety and to find strategies for coping. You may be seen on your own or with your family.

Occasionally, once you've tried a talking therapy, you might also be given a **medicine** to help if your anxiety problem has not got much better. A type of antidepressant is usually used.

Living with anxiety problems is difficult, but anxiety is treatable and doesn't have to keep making you unhappy.

Useful websites

⮑ **Anxiety UK**: www.anxietyuk.org.uk; a charity providing information and support for people with anxiety problems.

⮑ **YouthNet UK**: www.youthnet.org; online charity which guides and supports young people, enabling them to make informed choices, participate in society and achieve their ambitions.

Recommended reading

Other factsheets in this series:
Obsessive–compulsive disorder, CBT, Coping with stress, CAMHS, When bad things happen

Rays of Calm: Relaxation for Teenagers, by Christiane Kerr. This is a CD from the 'Calm for Kids' range created for teenagers. It talks through various relaxation techniques and visualisations designed to promote a sense of calm and well-being and to help teenagers deal with stress.

The Young Mind: An Essential Guide to Mental Health for Young Adults, Parents and Teachers, edited by Sue Bailey and Mike Shooter (2009) – an accessible, user-friendly handbook produced by the Royal College of Psychiatrists.

References

Baldwin DS, Anderson IM, Nutt DJ, et al. Evidence-based guidelines for the pharmacological treatment of anxiety disorders: recommendations from the British Association for Psychopharmacology. *J Psychopharmacol* 2005; 19: 567–96.

Green H, McGinnity A, Meltzer H, et al. *Mental Health of Children and Young People in Great Britain, 2004*. Office for National Statistics, 2005.

Ipser JC, Stein DJ, Hawkridge S, et al. Pharmacotherapy for anxiety disorders in children and adolescents. *Cochrane Database Syst Rev* 2009; 3: CD005170.

National Institute for Health and Clinical Excellence. *Anxiety: Guide to Self-Help Resources*. NICE, 2011.

O'Kearney RT, Anstey KJ, von Sanden C, et al. Behavioural and cognitive behavioural therapy for obsessive compulsive disorder in children and adolescents. *Cochrane Database Syst Rev* 2006; 4: CD004856.

Notes

15 Who's who in child and adolescent mental health services (CAMHS)

Information for young people

This is one in a series of factsheets for young people, with practical, up-to-date information about mental health problems (emotional, behavioural and psychiatric disorders) that can affect children and young people.

This factsheet describes who works in CAMHS, what they do and how they may be able to help if you or someone you know has a mental health problem.

Where can I find CAMHS?

Services in CAMHS are organised into four tiers. Many people when they talk about CAMHS mean tier 3 services – the community CAMHS teams. But CAMHS professionals can work in one or more of the following places:

- community CAMHS clinics (also called tier 3 services)
- out-patient clinics or alongside paediatricians in general hospitals
- specialised in-patient, day patient or out-patient units (tier 4 services)
- in schools and some GP practices (tier 2 services)
- alongside Social Services or youth offending services (YOS)
- in children's centres.

In addition to offering appointments in the above places, some CAMHS professionals can see you at home if it is difficult for you to meet elsewhere.

> ### What are CAMHS?
>
> Child and adolescent mental health services, in short called CAMHS, come in all shapes and sizes. They are made up of different mental health professionals, all working together to help young people and their families where there are mental health problems.

Who works in CAMHS?

The different child mental health professionals in the team usually include:

- **child and adolescent psychiatrists** – they are medically qualified doctors who specialise in working with young people with mental health problems and their families
- **clinical psychologists** – they can assess and help with children's psychological functioning, emotional well-being and development
- **child psychotherapists** – they are trained therapists who work with children helping to deal with their emotional and mental health problems
- **family therapists** – they are trained therapists who work with children and their families together to help them understand and manage the difficulties that are happening in their lives
- **social workers** – they are trained to help children and families who need extra support or help to keep them safe
- **mental health practitioners** – they are usually trained in mental health and help in the assessment (understanding) and management of emotional, behavioural and mental health problems.

Some teams can have other professionals such as paediatricians, educational psychologists, art therapists, and speech and language therapists.

All CAMHS professionals are trained and experienced in working with young people with mental health problems. They may also have some specialist skills, which they may use for specific conditions or treatments.

What problems can they help with?

Many children and young people are troubled by emotional, behavioural and psychiatric problems. These can cause worry and distress both to themselves and to those who care for them.

Professionals working in CAMHS deal with a wide range of mental health problems, including all those addressed in these factsheets and many more.

Liv, 15, talks about her experience of CAMHS

'I suppose I wasn't really me for quite a while before people noticed. In the end it was school; Mum and Dad were always far too busy to see what was really happening. I was being really short with everyone, teachers, even my friends; I fell out with quite a few people. I was picking fights, but I didn't know why. It was almost like it gave me an excuse to be able to shout and scream at someone.

My English teacher asked me to pop in to see our school nurse. After seeing me a few times, the nurse said she was worried about me and wanted me to see someone. She mentioned CAMHS. I didn't know what that meant; when she explained, I got quite cross. I told her I wasn't mad, I didn't need a shrink.

I went though, just to see if they would be any use. I met a doctor, a psychiatrist, first. But it wasn't like seeing any doctors I'd met before. We sat in chairs and had a really long talk. That was all. Then I went again and the same thing happened. Over a few weeks I managed to tell the doctor about what was going on at home; Mum and Dad, the arguing. She wondered about asking the whole family to come to a meeting.

They all came. The doctor was there, but she asked someone she works with, a family therapist, to join us too. They got my little sister to talk, which was amazing because she said she wouldn't say a thing. They got everyone to say something, somehow, without them really noticing. Mum was in tears when my sister said she didn't like seeing her so sad all the time. I was so relieved. They would really see now that it wasn't just me. It was all of us.' ✪

A large part of CAMHS professionals' work is to:

- identify the problem
- understand the causes
- advise about what may help.

Child psychiatrists are the only CAMHS professionals who can prescribe medication if it is needed. Sometimes, specially trained CAMHS nurses may prescribe for some illnesses (e.g. attention-deficit hyperactivity disorder (ADHD)). Other CAMHS professionals, for example child psychotherapists, psychologists and family therapists, are particularly skilled in providing talking therapies of different sorts. Most of the work that they do with children, young people and their families is done through out-patient appointments, while the young person continues to live at home.

Child and adolescent mental health professionals are sometimes asked to provide expert opinion to the courts about child welfare issues.

How can I be seen in CAMHS?

Your GP, health visitor, paediatrician, school doctor or nurse, educational psychologist, special educational needs coordinating officer (SENCO) in school, or social worker will be able to discuss any concerns and arrange for an appointment in a CAMHS clinic, if necessary.

Useful website

⮕ **Young Minds**: www.youngminds.org.uk; a charity committed to improving the emotional well-being and mental health of children and young people.

Recommended reading

CAMHS Inside Out: A Young Person's Guide to Child and Adolescent Mental Health Services. A downloadable booklet and a leaflet to tell young people more about what to expect from CAMHS. It has been prepared by the Royal College of Psychiatrists and is available on our website (www.rcpsych.ac.uk/quality/qualityandaccreditation/qinmaccamhs/youngpersonsguidetocamhs.aspx).

Reference

Department of Health. Standard 9: The Mental Health and Psychological Well-Being of Children and Young People. Department of Health, 2004.

Notes

....

....

....

1 Good parenting

Information for parents, carers and anyone who works with young people

This is one in a series of factsheets for parents, teachers and anyone who works with young people, with practical, up-to-date information about mental health problems (emotional, behavioural and psychiatric disorders) that can affect children and young people.

This factsheet looks at why it is important to use good parenting skills from an early age. It also gives practical tips on some of the best ways to discipline a child, while maintaining a happy, healthy relationship with them.

Why is parenting important?

Setting limits (rules) is an important part of everyday life. Rules make it possible for us to get along with one another. If children do not learn how to behave, they will find it difficult to get on, both with grown-ups and with other children. They will find it hard to learn at school, will misbehave and will probably become unhappy and frustrated.

What helps?

It is important to make sure that children feel secure, loved and valued, and that all adults looking after them notice when they are behaving well. The trick to this is to find strategies that work well for you and your child. Here are some ideas.

- **Be consistent**

  Try to say the same thing each time. Be clear about the rules you want to stick to. If you don't stick to the rules and give in, then the next time you try to set limits, your child is likely to play up even more because they have learnt that you will probably give in again.

- **Give lots of praise**

  Let your child know when they have done something well and when you are pleased with them. Be specific so that the child knows which behaviour you are wanting to encourage. For example, give them a hug or a kiss, tell them how great they are doing and point out the good behaviour. You need to do this straight away at the time when you see the behaviour you want to encourage.

- **Plan ahead**

  It helps if you and your child know the rules for particular situations before they happen. Don't make them up as you go along (e.g. if bedtime is 7.00 pm, make sure you both stick to it).

- **Involve your child**

  Sit down with your child and talk to them about good behaviour. You might be surprised about how much you both agree on.

- **Be calm**

  This can be difficult in the heat of the moment, but it does help if you can be calm and clear with the words you use, for example 'Please switch off the TV' or 'It's bedtime'.

- **Be clear with your child**

  For example, 'Please put your toys away' tells your child exactly what you want them to do. Simply telling them to 'be good' will not help them know what behaviour you are expecting. If your child can't understand you, they can't cooperate with you. So it is best to keep instructions brief and positive.

- **Be realistic**

  It's no good promising a wonderful reward or threatening to remove their favourite activity if you can't keep to your word. It is much better to offer small rewards rather than punishments. For example, 'When you have tidied your room, you can have an ice cream'. Don't expect too much too soon. Change usually takes time. For this reason expect to progress in small steps. So if your child has started to or partly tidied their room, praise them for what they have done: 'Well done for putting those toys in the box'.

What does it mean to be a good parent?

Parenting is an important part of loving and caring for your child. Good parenting is about providing a warm, secure home life, helping your child to learn the rules of life (e.g. how to share, respect others) and to develop good self-esteem. You may have to stop them from doing things they shouldn't be doing, but it is just as important to encourage them to do the things you do want them to do.

> **Janet, mother of Sam (6)**
>
> 'When Sam's dad and I separated, I had big problems getting Sam to be in bed for 7 pm. At first he was upset at night and did not want to go to bed until I did. After the school holidays when he started year 1 I decided he should go to bed at a regular time but he refused, threw himself on the floor, cried and shouted.
>
> My GP said that children seem to manage better with regular routines. Sam and I started a sort of routine; he has a story in bed and I sit with him for a while and then he falls asleep. Of course it's different when Sam sleeps in his dad's flat. His dad says he doesn't have any problems, but it's at weekends and not a school night, so he's allowed to stay up and watch TV.
>
> When Sam spends weekends with me he wants to stay up, but I am sticking to 7 pm on Sundays because he has school the next day. It's hard to be firm but there are fewer rows now as Sam knows I will not give in.' ✪

The importance of your relationship

Everybody can at times feel cross and upset. It is helpful if you do spend some time together doing nice things. It is easier to do this if it is already a part of your everyday life. So try to plan for some good times together every day or most days. For example, you could plan to play a game, read together or cook with your child even for 10 minutes.

How not to let it go wrong

- **Be clear and consistent**

  Your own experience of childhood is very important. Even if you want to do things differently from your own experience, you may find yourself doing the same with your own children. Or you find that you are doing the opposite! It is helpful if you can aim to be as clear and consistent as you can be.

- **Show a unified front**

  If parents disagree about rules and their expectations for their children, the children may get mixed up because they don't know what they are expected to do. They may find that if they ask each parent/carer the same question they get different answers. So, whether parents are together or living in different homes, it is important, as far as possible, that everyone who cares for the child agrees on the most important matters and the behaviours they want to encourage their children to do.

- **Encourage positive behaviours**

  Parenting can be hard work, both physically and emotionally. It is easy to let things slip if you are stressed, depressed, tired, very busy or don't have any help looking after your children. Without consistent encouragement and expectations, children may develop bad habits with their behaviour.

Where can I get help?

Talking problems over with other parents or friends is often useful. Talk to your child's teachers, as there may be a similar problem at school. It will help your child if you and the teachers work together to agree on how to tackle the problem. Changing a child's behaviour can be a slow process, but it can be done.

You can ask your health visitor, school or practice nurse for advice. Some parents/carers may find attending their local family centre or joining a parenting programme helpful.

If more specialist help is needed, you may refer to the local child and adolescent mental health service (CAMHS). Specialists can help you work out what the problem might be and suggest practical ways of helping.

Recommended reading

Other factsheets in this series: Restless and excitable child, CAMHS

The Young Mind: An Essential Guide to Mental Health for Young Adults, Parents and Teachers, edited by Sue Bailey and Mike Shooter (2009) – an accessible, user-friendly handbook produced by the Royal College of Psychiatrists.

Understanding Your Child's Behaviour: Information for Families – a booklet produced by Contact a Family, focuses on children with a disability.

References

Kane GA, Wood VA, Barlow J. Parenting programmes: a systematic review and synthesis of qualitative research. *Child Care Health Dev* 2007; 33: 784–93.

Rutter M, Bishop D, Pine D, et al (eds) *Rutter's Child and Adolescent Psychiatry* (5th edn). Wiley–Blackwell, 2008.

Scott S. An update on interventions for conduct disorder. *Adv Psychiatr Treat* 2008; 14: 61–70.

Useful websites

- ➲ **Family Lives**: http://familylives.org.uk; help and advice to parents bringing up children and teenagers. Helpline: 0808 800 2222.
- ➲ **Positive Parenting**: www.parenting.org.uk; a useful website offering training, resources and literature.
- ➲ **Patient.co.uk**: www.patient.co.uk; information and links on various difficulties and conditions.
- ➲ **Young Minds**: www.youngminds.org.uk; for any adult concerned about the emotions and behaviour of a child or young person. Parents' helpline: 0808 802 5544.

Notes

2 The restless and excitable child
Information for parents, carers and anyone who works with young people

This is one in a series of factsheets for parents, teachers and anyone who works with young people, with practical, up-to-date information about mental health problems (emotional, behavioural and psychiatric disorders) that can affect children and young people.

This factsheet looks at why some children are more restless and excitable than others, gives advice about how to deal with an overactive child, and suggests where to go to get extra help if you feel you are unable to cope on your own.

What makes children overactive?

There are many things that can make a child overactive. The following should give you some guidance as to the reasons for your child's behaviour. Finding the reasons may help you to come up with some solutions to deal with them.

- **Being a parent**

  If parents are unhappy, depressed or worried, they tend to pay less attention to their children. They may find they can't spend the time they need to help children play constructively, or they may find that when they do play with them, they spend a lot of time telling them to be quiet. Children learn from this that they have to be naughty or noisy to get any attention from their mum or dad.

- **No clear rules**

  It is important to have simple rules about what is allowed and what is not. If two parents are involved, they both need to agree about the rules, and be consistent and fair when they say 'no'. This will help the child to know what is expected and to learn self-control.

- **Child's temperament**

  We are all born with different temperaments. Some children are livelier, noisier and more outgoing than others. They may prefer going out and being with other people than quietly reading a book or playing with toys by themselves. Quite often, children who are active like this are also excitable and may go over the top while playing. Although this can be a nuisance, it is nothing to worry about, but you may need some help in finding ways to help your child calm down.

- **Learning and other problems**

  Some children find it hard to learn things that other children find easy. They may need special help at school. They may seem quite young for their age and find it hard to concentrate on work or control their behaviour as well as other children.

- **ADHD**

  Some children may be affected by attention-deficit hyperactivity disorder (ADHD). If this is the case, seek help.

- **Hearing problems**

  Glue ear (ear infections) is a common example of a hearing problem. If a child has glue ear, they will find it hard to hear what other people say, will tend to shout and may want the television turned up very loudly.

- **Food**

  Some children do seem to react to certain foods by becoming restless and irritable. This is not as common as some people think, but occasionally it can be a real problem.

What is meant by an 'overactive child'?

Young children are often restless and excitable. Their noisy liveliness is usually just a part of being young. Although it may be tiring, it is usually nothing to worry about.

Sometimes youngsters may be so active and noisy that it makes life difficult for their parents and other children. A child like this may be demanding and excitable, and chatter away nineteen to the dozen. They may be noisy, may not do as they are told, and will probably find it difficult to sit still. Adults may say that the child is 'hyperactive', but the trouble with this word is that professionals use it to describe extreme and sometimes dangerous behaviour, such as running out into a busy road.

Kate talks about her 7-year-old son, Ron

'Ron was my first son. He was always a lively, energetic child, even as a toddler – early to walk and run. I could not keep up the pace and would feel exhausted running after him. It drove me nuts. When he was 6, I met Linda, his classmate's mum. She told me she had the same difficulties with her son, but then she attended a parenting group and it was really helpful. She said it took some time, but it was really basic and it made all the difference. I agreed to give it a try. At first I didn't think the group was for me as I found it difficult to talk to strangers about my difficulties controlling my child … but soon it was OK. All the parents had had similar experiences. Just talking to others made it feel much easier. I was not shouting at Ron "stop it" all the time. I was more tolerant, I praised him when he ate his breakfast and gave him a hug. It seemed all calmer, even Ron seemed to notice the difference. He seemed a happier child, listening to me. When I wanted him to really do something, I would just look at him, speak to him calmly and tell him what to do, in simple words. No long explanations. Just a few words and it worked. So simple. Ron loves his evening time before tea on his bike while I walk the dog. I feel it has worked out well … just in time.' ✪

Useful websites

➲ **Family Lives**: http://familylives.org.uk; help and advice to parents bringing up children and teenagers. Helpline: 0808 800 2222.

➲ **Positive Parenting**: www.parenting.org.uk; useful website offering training, resources and literature for parents and those who work with children.

How can I get my child to calm down?

Try to make sure you spend time with your child on their own, so that they know you are interested in them. This will give you the chance to plan and praise.

- **Plan**

  Spend time with your children doing something they enjoy. Get into a routine and plan what they are going to be doing for the day or the weekend. It is helpful to arrange to have friends to come and play (encouraging their social development), and it gives you a break when they are invited back! It is also helpful to engage children in regular activities such as football or trampoline sessions, cubs, Brownies, etc. because this gives you a chance to meet other parents who can provide an informal support network. You can also make clear times when you expect them to play quietly on their own.

- **Praise**

  Take every opportunity to praise your child. Be as clear as possible. It is vital that they understand exactly what they have done to please you. For example, 'You've been playing so quietly on your own … what a good boy you are!' or 'What a good footballer you are!'

Where can I get help?

Lively, excitable behaviour is a common problem for parents. Your health visitor will be used to giving advice about this. If there seems to be a problem with your child's hearing or if there seems to be a reaction to foods, your GP should be able to help and refer to a specialist if required. If they think that the child might have a learning difficulty or a hyperactivity disorder, they will refer you to a clinical psychologist, paediatrician or child and adolescent mental health service (CAMHS).

Recommended reading

Other factsheets in this series:
Good parenting, Behavioural problems and conduct disorder, General learning disability, ADHD, CAMHS

Parenting Pre-School Children: How to Cope with Common Behavioural Problems, by Paul Stallard, is a useful and practical book. Published by How to Books, 1998.

The Incredible Years: A Troubleshooting Guide for Parents of Children Aged 3 to 8, by Carolyn Webster-Stratton. Umbrella Press, 1992.

References

Bailey S, Shooter M (eds) *The Young Mind: An Essential Guide to Mental Health for Young Adults, Parents and Teachers*. RCPsych Publications, 2009.

Rutter M, Bishop D, Pine D, et al (eds) *Rutter's Child and Adolescent Psychiatry* (5th edn). Wiley–Blackwell, 2008.

For a catalogue of public education materials or copies of our leaflets contact: Book Sales/Leaflets, The Royal College of Psychiatrists, 17 Belgrave Square, London SW1X 8PG. Email: leaflets@rcpsych.ac.uk, tel: 020 7235 2351 ext. 6146.

Revised by the Royal College of Psychiatrists' Child and Family Public Education Editorial Board. With grateful thanks to Dr Kate Gingell. This leaflet reflects the best possible evidence at the time of writing.
The Royal College of Psychiatrists is a charity registered in England and Wales (228636) and in Scotland (SC038369).
© The Royal College of Psychiatrists 2013

3 Dealing with tantrums
Information for parents, carers and anyone who works with young people

This is one in a series of factsheets for parents, teachers and anyone who works with young people, with practical, up-to-date information about mental health problems (emotional, behavioural and psychiatric disorders) that can affect children and young people.

This factsheet explains why children may have tantrums and gives some practical tips about how to deal with them.

What causes a tantrum?

This is a normal part of growing up. Between the ages of 1 and 4 years, most children will have tantrums. As children grow they are learning to become more physically independent. For example, they may want to play, want to dress and feed themselves, or pour their own juice. Your child therefore can get very upset if they are unable to do something or if they are stopped. A battle between freedom and frustration can lead to tantrums.

> **What is a tantrum?**
>
> A tantrum is usually a short period of angry outburst or unreasonable behaviour such as crying, screaming, shouting and throwing objects.

Tantrums can also occur when a child is:

- tired
- hungry
- feeling ignored
- worried or anxious – a younger child may be unable to tell you that they are anxious and they may cry, become clingy and have tantrums.

What can I do when my child is having a tantrum?

Your child's screams and yells can be alarming. You may feel angry, discouraged and hopeless. You will almost certainly be embarrassed if a tantrum occurs in a public place or in front of other people.

It is not easy being a parent or carer of a toddler. However, it is important to set the rules, so your child learns to deal with their emotions. Remember, it is only natural that children will try to push the limits. Here are some ideas which may work for you and your child.

- **Don't panic**

  The main thing to do is to stay calm and not to get upset. Just remind yourself that this is normal, that lots of parents do deal with it, be reassured that you will manage this too.

- **Ignore the tantrum**

  You should calmly continue with whatever you are doing – chatting to someone else, packing your shopping or whatever. Every so often check to make sure your child is safe. Ignoring your child is very hard, but if you answer back, or even smack them, you are giving them the attention they are demanding.

- **Be consistent with rules**

  You are trying to teach your child that rules are important and that you will stick to them.

- **Pay attention to any good behaviour**

  As soon as you see any signs of calming down, e.g. they stop screaming, praise them. Turn your full attention back to the child, talk to them with warmth and admiration. If you reward the new behaviour like this, your child is more likely to stay calm and carry on being good.

What can I do to prevent temper tantrums?

Planning ahead can help to avoid a tantrum, if you know when they are likely to occur or notice a pattern your child shows before having a tantrum. Here are some examples:

- manage boredom when in a waiting room by taking their favourite books and toys to the doctor's surgery with you
- storing their favourite biscuits out of sight, rather than where they can see them

- manage a tired child by giving them an afternoon nap, instead of staying awake all day
- manage hunger by offering a snack after nursery at 3.30 pm, instead of having to wait until 5.00 pm for tea
- distraction can help – you may be able to avoid a tantrum by diverting your child's attention.

Where can I get help?

Talking problems over with other parents, family or friends is often useful. Talk to your child's teachers, as there may be a similar problem at nursery or school.

If this does not help and the tantrums are getting you down, ask your health visitor, school, practice nurse or general practitioner for advice. Many parents and carers find parenting programmes like Triple P (www.triplep.net) or Webster Stratton groups (www.incredibleyears.com) helpful. Sometimes more specialist help from child and adolescent mental health services (CAMHS) may be required, especially when there are other worrying difficulties for the child, or when tantrums occur too long and often, with child hurting themself or others.

Useful websites

⊃ **Young Minds**: www.youngminds.org.uk; for any adult concerned about the emotions and behaviour of a child or young person. Parents' helpline: 0808 802 5544.

⊃ **HandsOnScotland**: www.handonscotland.co.uk; a website with a toolkit of helpful responses to encourage children and young people's emotional well-being.

Recommended reading

Other factsheets in this series:
Good parenting, CAMHS

References

Bailey S, Shooter M (eds) *The Young Mind: An Essential Guide to Mental Health for Young Adults, Parents and Teachers*. RCPsych Publications, 2009.

Rutter M, Bishop D, Pine D, et al (eds) *Rutter's Child and Adolescent Psychiatry* (5th edn). Wiley–Blackwell, 2008.

Hannah talks about having a child with tantrums

'My son, Dylan, was about 22 months' old when he started banging his head, screaming and crying when he really wanted something and I wasn't able to give it to him straight away.

Some members of the family said that it was because Dylan was becoming more independent and that he was testing boundaries. Martin, my fiancé, used to give in to Dylan really easily, and we would often disagree with how to manage his behaviour in public and would argue about it.

It was really stressful and embarrassing when Dylan would take things off the shelves at the supermarket and start screaming when I took them away because they were not safe.

When he started banging his head against the floor, I was really surprised. He had never done anything like this before and I was really worried that he might harm himself badly. I soon realised that Dylan was okay and behaved better if I stayed calm when he threw a tantrum, and would settle down if I didn't pay too much attention to his behaviour. I also noticed that Dylan would be well behaved for longer if I rewarded his good behaviour and said lots of positive things to him about how well he was doing. We started taking Dylan to the swimming pool which he really liked too and he soon grew out of the head-banging.' ✪

Notes

....

....

....

For a catalogue of public education materials or copies of our leaflets contact: Book Sales/Leaflets, The Royal College of Psychiatrists, 17 Belgrave Square, London SW1X 8PG. Email: leaflets@rcpsych.ac.uk, tel: 020 7235 2351 ext. 6146.

Revised by the Royal College of Psychiatrists' Child and Family Public Education Editorial Board. With grateful thanks to Dr Fareeha Amber Sadiq. This leaflet reflects the best possible evidence at the time of writing.
The Royal College of Psychiatrists is a charity registered in England and Wales (228636) and in Scotland (SC038369). © The Royal College of Psychiatrists 2013

4 Children who soil or wet themselves
Information for parents, carers and anyone who works with young people

This is one in a series of factsheets for parents, teachers and anyone who works with young people, with practical, up-to-date information about mental health problems (emotional, behavioural and psychiatric disorders) that can affect children and young people.

This factsheet looks at why why children may soil or wet themselves and offers some practical advice about how to cope with this problem.

What causes bed-wetting?

There are several reasons why children may still wet the bed after the age of 5.

- Some children may just develop slower or may not yet be able to wake themselves up when their bladders are full.
- Children are more likely to wet their bed if they are very tired and sleeping deeply. Some children who are normally dry may wet their bed when this happens or when unwell.
- Bed-wetting is more likely to happen when children drink a lot before they go to bed. Their bladder may not be able to hold all the urine that is produced and empty without them waking up.
- For some children, where they have been dry for a period of time, bed-wetting can be a sign of emotional distress. They may be experiencing anxiety or stress, or it may be a reaction to major changes in their life (such as when a new baby arrives in the family or when they start school).
- Bed-wetting may also be caused by constipation, urinary tract infection (UTI) or lack of a hormone called 'vasopressin'.
- Children are more likely to experience bed-wetting if one or both of their parents had wet the bed as children too.

What are the effects of bed-wetting?

Bed-wetting may mean that your child misses out on sleepovers, holidays or trips away. They may feel embarrassed or ashamed that they still wet the bed. This can affect their self-esteem.

Parents/carers rarely talk about their children wetting the bed. This may be because people often think that their child is the only one with a problem. It may also be because they feel guilty or responsible that they haven't been able to do something about the problem.

Is it deliberate or due to laziness?

Bed-wetting is an involuntary loss of urine at night when a child is sleeping. This means it is an accident and it is not their fault. You should never blame your child. Making your child feel bad, ashamed or anxious will only make the problem harder to deal with.

What can I do?

Below are some things that you can try out initially.

- Make sure your child drinks normally until about an hour before they go to bed. After this, allow small mouthfuls of water to relieve thirst. Avoid fizzy or caffeine-based drinks as these will stimulate the kidneys and lead to more urine being produced.
- Ensure that going to the toilet is part of your child's bedtime routine every night. Encourage them to sit long enough to fully empty their bladder.

What is bed-wetting?

'Enuresis' is a term used for wetting or passing of urine without control at an age when it would be expected. This can occur either during the day or night.

Bed-wetting (also called 'nocturnal enuresis') is when a child passes urine when asleep at night. Bed-wetting is normal in children under 2 years of age. Most children will develop night-time dryness between 2 and 5 years of age, but some may still wet the bed during this time.

If your child reaches the age of 6 and is still regularly wetting the bed, this is known as 'primary enuresis'. If your child starts to wet the bed after a period of being dry (e.g. for 6 months), this is known as 'secondary enuresis'. In either case, you should seek advice.

- You may sometimes find it helpful to lift your child from their bed and sit them on the toilet. Older children may try waking themselves up.
- Make sure that you praise and encourage your child's steps towards dry nights – tell them 'well done' for any dry nights. This often helps.
- Set up a positive reward system for behaviour that is likely to contribute to night-time dryness, without focusing on the actual bed-wetting. For example, rewards may be given for: drinking recommended levels of fluid during the day, using the toilet to pass urine before going to bed/sleep, engaging in management (e.g. taking medication or helping to change the sheets).

What if it doesnt get better?

If bed-wetting continues and you don't see an increase in dry nights, you should seek advice from your GP, school nurse or family health visitor. They will be able to offer you support and advice, and to refer your child to a specialist such as paediatrician or continence nurse, if they feel this is appropriate.

If the bed-wetting started after your child had been dry at night for a period of time (secondary enuresis), and physical problems have been ruled out, your GP or school nurse might suggest that you see someone from your local child and adolescent mental health service (CAMHS).

What other treatments are available?

It is important to reward agreed positive behaviour (e.g. changing the sheets rather than just dry nights) along with applying treatments described below.

- Bell and pad

   The 'enuresis alarm' is a pad that is connected to an electrical buzzer. When your child starts to wet the bed, the buzzer goes off. This should wake your child who then gets up to go to the toilet. Gradually, your child will recognise the sensation of a full bladder and learn to wake by themselves when it is full. It may take your child weeks or months to become completely dry at night. To be successful, your child must be motivated to become dry at night and be fully involved with the process.

- Medication

   Sometimes children may be prescribed medication by their GP or specialist clinic. The medications work by either relaxing the bladder so it can expand and hold more urine, or help the kidneys produce less urine.

Daytime wetting

Daytime wetting affects about 1 in 75 children over the age of 5 and is more common in girls. It can occur by itself or when a child is also bed-wetting. This problem can be very stressful or embarrassing for children when they go to school as it may lead to teasing or bullying.

Emily, 7, with bed-wetting

'Emily developed night-time dryness at around age 4. Despite being dry for many years, following the birth of her baby brother, she regularly wet the bed at night (this is known as "secondary enuresis"). Her parents felt very stressed and angry about this and viewed this behaviour as being lazy, attention-seeking and defiant. They responded by shouting and criticising her. In response, Emily tried to cover up her wet bedclothes and seemed more withdrawn and quieter than normal.

Physical causes were ruled out. The parents were told that a setback in normal development, when previously dry, was more likely to be a reaction to psychological (or in some cases physical) stress, i.e. the arrival of a new baby, rather than being caused by laziness, attention-seeking or defiance.

The family limited Emily's intake of fluids before bedtime, particularly fizzy and caffeinated drinks. She was encouraged to have a routine when going to the toilet before bedtime. To help reinforce bladder control, she was encouraged to change her own nightwear and bedding, following episodes of wetting. Praise and encouragement were given to Emily by her parents for steps taken towards dry nights. A reward system was set up for her. She could earn rewards for performing activities, such as going to the toilet before bedtime each night and taking responsibility for changing her wet nightwear and bedding.

To help Emily adjust to having a new brother, her parents also spent time with her each day engaged in some positive activities, such as playing and talking. To help her feel more involved, she was also given some specific jobs to help with the care of the baby.' ✪

What causes it?

A variety of physical or emotional reasons can cause daytime wetting. Younger children in particular may be so busy playing or doing their work that they simply forget to use the toilet or leave it too late. They may also be in a hurry when going to the toilet and do not completely empty their bladder.

Some children may be constipated and this can put pressure on the bladder, or have an UTI that needs medical treatment. It can also happen if your child is anxious or has experienced emotional upset.

What can help?

Encourage your child to **drink about 6–8 glasses** of water-based drinks such as cordials or squashes throughout the day, as this helps the bladder to fill properly. It is also important to encourage **healthy eating** to avoid any constipation.

Parents can set up a **toilet routine**, with set toilet times to discourage 'holding on' or forgetting to go to the toilet. Children may need regular reminders to go to the toilet, or they can be given a timer or a vibrating wristwatch to remind them to go to the toilet regularly. To increase a child's motivation to go to the toilet regularly, set up a 'star chart' with small **rewards** for going to the toilet and for dry pants at the end of the day.

If accidents do happen, **try not to get angry**, shout or use punishments. This is likely to add to any shame or embarrassment that the child may already feel and raise their anxiety, all of which are likely to make the problem worse.

Speak to your GP or school nurse if difficulties persist as they can refer you to a specialist if necessary.

Soiling

Soiling (encopresis) occurs when a child does not reliably use the toilet for a poo/bowel motion. They may dirty their pants or go to the toilet in inappropriate places.

This is normal in toddlers and younger children as they learn to control their bowels in the toilet. However, if it is having a negative effect on family life, you may wish to seek additional support. Under normal circumstances, healthy children will develop control over their bowels by the age of 4.

What causes it?

There can be a number of different reasons that affect a child's ability to go to the toilet for a poo.

- Not learning a regular toilet routine is a common cause of soiling. The child may be reluctant to use the toilet. This may sometimes be part of a general pattern of behaviour where a child refuses to do what you want them to.

- Sometimes a change in diet, an infection, taking medication or life events, such as a house move, starting nursery or another change within the family, can trigger constipation.

- Severe constipation causes the bowel to be blocked with hard poo. The child finds it painful to pass this hard poo, and so becomes more constipated. Liquid poo then leaks around the blockage, staining clothes. Children who are constipated may become irritable, with a lack of energy and a loss of appetite.

Jack, 6, with soiling

'Jack's parents felt he was a "picky eater" from a very young age, preferring crisps, coke, chips and processed cheese. Jack became constipated and his poo became dry and hard to pass. When Jack tried to poo, it was very painful.

Jack became fearful of going to the toilet so he hung on. His poo became increasingly hard and stuck in his bowel, causing liquid faeces to trickle around the blockage and causing him to soil his pants. Jack was very ashamed, and hid his pants in many different places. This caused lots of arguments between him and his dad. His dad shouted at him to go to the toilet. Jack became reluctant to cooperate with his parents. He became quite grumpy and pale.

Jack's treatment focused on moving the blocked, dry stools with medication prescribed by his GP. He was encouraged to drink water and eat healthy foods, with a very simple reward chart.

Jack's school nurse advised his mum to make the toilet a rewarding place, by allowing him a special comic or game he could only use when he was practising pooing. His parents were also given some information on constipation and soiling.

Jack's dad worked at reducing the conflict around Jack's toileting routine by reinforcing "trying to poo", rather than passing a poo. They praised him for taking medication and rewarded him with family days out.

Jack's soiling improved and his family felt relieved and positive about each other.' ✪

- Sometimes a child links pain with pooing. They are fearful and try to hold in their poo, making it even harder and difficult to pass. This happens when a child in the past has had hard poo in the bowel, which caused a small split in the anus called a 'fissure' that is extremely painful.

What can help?

- If your child is soiling because they have never had a toileting routine, you can help by encouraging them to establish a regular **routine** by praising them for their effort and any successes. You can ask for support from your health visitor or school nurse with this. **Star charts** and stickers can prove motivating for children. Ensure that any of your responses are **not punishing**.

- If you suspect your child is constipated or their poo is painful to pass, it is a good idea to visit your GP. They may recommend **medication** to help clear your child's bowel. Alongside this, you can help by making sure that they eat a lot of fruit, vegetables and foods high in fibre, as well as exercising and drinking lots of water. This will make the poo softer and easier to pass. Again, toileting routines, star charts and non-punishing responses can be helpful.

- If your child is not constipated, the cause may be emotional or psychological. If they start to soil or to smear faeces after no previous difficulties, they may be **emotionally upset**. If you can find out what is upsetting them and sort it out, the soiling may then improve. If it carries on, your GP may suggest specialist help from the local CAMHS.

Recommended reading

Other factsheets in this series: Sleep problems in childhood and adolescence, Behavioural problems and conduct disorder, CAMHS

Daytime Wetting in Childhood – A Helpful Guide for Parents and Carers, by P. Dobson. Published by ERIC, 2006.

References

National Institute for Health and Clinical Excellence. *Diagnosis and Management of Idiopathic Childhood Constipation in Primary and Secondary Care* (CG99). NICE, 2010.

National Institute for Health and Clinical Excellence. *The Management of Bedwetting and Nocturnal Enuresis in Children and Young People* (CG111). NICE, 2010.

Rutter M, Bishop D, Pine D, et al (eds) *Rutter's Child and Adolescent Psychiatry* (5th edn). Wiley–Blackwell, 2008.

Wells M, Bonner L. *Effective Management of Bladder and Bowel Problems in Children.* Class Publishing, 2008.

Useful websites

- ⮞ **ERIC (Education and Resources for Improving Childhood continence)**: www.eric.org.uk; information and advice about day and night wetting for parents, young people and professionals.

- ⮞ **NHS Choices**: www.nhs.uk; information on day and night wetting and soiling.

- ⮞ **HandsOnScotland**: www.handsonscotland.co.uk; practical information, tools and activities to respond helpfully to troubling behaviour and to help children and young people to flourish.

Notes

For a catalogue of public education materials or copies of our leaflets contact: Book Sales/Leaflets, The Royal College of Psychiatrists, 17 Belgrave Square, London SW1X 8PG. Email: leaflets@rcpsych.ac.uk, tel: 020 7235 2351 ext. 6146.

Revised by the Royal College of Psychiatrists' Child and Family Public Education Editorial Board. With grateful thanks to Dr Beverley Dayus, Dr Lindsey Hampson and Emma Ridoch. This leaflet reflects the best possible evidence at the time of writing.

5 Sleep problems in childhood and adolescence
Information for parents, carers and anyone who works with young people

This is one in a series of factsheets for parents, teachers and anyone who works with young people, with practical, up-to-date information about mental health problems (emotional, behavioural and psychiatric disorders) that can affect children and young people.

This factsheet looks at why some children and young people have sleep problems, and offers some practical advice on how to deal with them.

How much sleep does a child need?

The amount of sleep needed gradually decreases from infancy to adulthood. Every child is different but as a general rule of thumb:

- toddlers need about 12–14 hours' sleep (including daytime naps)
- pre-schoolers (aged 3–5) need 11–12 hours' sleep
- school-age children need 10–11 hours' sleep
- teenagers need 9–10 hours' sleep.

Why can't my child sleep?

There can be different reasons.

- Very young children often fear being left alone at night. This is called 'separation anxiety' and is normal at a young age.
- Bedtime fears – many young children are afraid of the dark.
- Bad habits – napping too much during the day.
- 'I'm not sleepy' – you might find that when your child gets very tired, they get irritable, aggressive or even overactive (hence the phrase 'overtired').

Daytime sleepiness

This can simply be caused by your child not getting enough sleep at night. They could be going to bed too late or having problems sleeping, for reasons described above.

There are a number of less common reasons for daytime sleepiness.

- **Large tonsils and adenoids** at the back and sides of the throat can cause breathing difficulties that can wake a child many times each night. The child may not remember waking up, but you may notice that they snore loudly and sleep restlessly. This is called obstructive sleep apnoea. An operation to remove the tonsils and adenoids may be needed.
- **Restless legs syndrome** is a condition where the child complains of crawling feelings or 'growing pains' in their legs that make them want to keep moving them, which stops them getting to sleep.
- **Narcolepsy** is an unusual condition that causes unpredictable attacks of sleep during the day. People with narcolepsy may also have sudden attacks of weakness – this is called **cataplexy**.
- In teenagers, **drug or alcohol misuse** is sometimes a factor.
- Some young people who have **depression** sleep more than usual.

Nightmares

Most children have nightmares occasionally. These are vivid and frightening dreams. Children will usually remember the dream, and will need to be comforted so that they can get back to sleep.

Nightmares can also be caused by worry, nasty accidents, bullying and abuse of any kind. You can help by encouraging your child to talk about the dream or draw a picture of it. This will help you to find out the cause of the upset and work out what help or support your child needs.

What does it mean when a child has sleep problems?

One of the most common problems in toddlers and young children is sleeplessness. The child may have difficulty settling to sleep, or wakes in the night and wants a parent.

Teenagers can also have problems with sleeplessness. They might find it hard to sleep if they are worried, drink too much tea or coffee, cola or energy drinks, or use illegal drugs. Some will just get into the habit of going to sleep very late. After a while, they find that they can't get to sleep at an earlier time.

Sometimes, difficulty in sleeping is part of depression.

Night terrors

Night terrors most commonly affect children between the ages of 4 and 12 years. They are completely different from nightmares or anxiety-related dreams.

Unlike nightmares, night terrors happen to young children an hour or two after falling asleep. The first sign is that your child is screaming uncontrollably and seems to be awake. In spite of appearances, your child is still asleep. They will not be able to recognise you, will be confused and unable to communicate, and it is usually hard to reassure them. It is best not to try and wake them, but sit with them until the night terror passes, usually after about 5 minutes. Try not to feel upset yourself. It can be very distressing to see your child so disturbed, but they will not remember it in the morning. Children usually grow out of this.

Sleepwalking

Sleepwalking is similar to night terrors, but instead of being terrified, the child gets up out of bed and moves around. The main thing you can do to help is to make sure that they don't hurt themselves. You may need to take practical precautions, like using a stair-gate, making sure that windows and doors are securely locked, and that fires are screened or put out. This is also something that children tend to grow out of.

Why sleep problems matter

Sleep problems are very common. Most children's sleep problems happen only occasionally. They are not serious and get better on their own, with time. If they don't, you need to take them seriously. As well as being upsetting, they may interfere with your child's learning and behaviour. There may be underlying physical or mental health problems.

What can I do to help my child sleep better?

It is important that your child has a regular sleep routine.

- Decide on **regular times** for going to bed and getting up, and stick to these times.

- Develop a consistent, relaxing **bedtime routine** with your child. This should start with quiet time to help your child to wind down; for example, a bath followed by a short bedtime story before you say goodnight. This helps children to settle, and should end with your child falling asleep without the need for you to be with them.

- It is important to **be loving, but firm**, about when it is time for your child to settle down for the night. When your child cries out, it is important to be sure that they are not wet, ill or in pain. It is best to do this quickly, while still comforting and reassuring them. Don't spend too much time with them or take them into your bed, because this will reward them for being awake.

- A **dummy** can help to comfort young infants who wake needing to suck. Once you have weaned your child on to solid foods, it is best not to give them a bottle or dummy at night – if they wake and can't find it, they will probably start crying. A cuddly toy or favourite blanket can often help young children to cope with their separation anxiety.

Jason, 15, talks about his problems with sleeping

'I never liked high school. I got named "junky boy" on the first day. I have diabetes… I started doing my own injections in high school and had to wear a special wristband. It didn't take long for the bullying to get worse. I stopped going out and spent more time alone.

At home I spent a lot of my time in my room on the computer staying up late. I started to feel really tired in the morning, and soon I wouldn't get up and refused to go to school.

I felt "ill" all the time and my brother started to call me "vampire". I looked pale and had no friends. My parents had had enough of trying to get me to school and I even remember seeing Mum in tears. That was when we spoke to the nurse in the diabetic clinic and it was suggested that I go to see the psychiatry team in hospital. I was reluctant, but I did go and I'm really glad.

When we met the team, we talked about my problems and I was asked to keep a sleep diary. We also tried "sleep hygiene techniques" – these are tips on helping you sleep. This meant making changes to my eating, exercise and spending time on my computer. At first this led to more arguments with my family. Later we were able to go back and talk about this with the practitioner. It seemed a long time but after a few weeks, my sleep was better.

I now have a work placement and was lucky to get involved with a group doing activities with young people who have similar problems to me. I met my girlfriend there.

I am sleeping much better now and go to the special teenage diabetic clinic where I get more support. My mum is smiling for the first time in months.' ✪

How can I help a teenager sleep better?

- Agree with them reasonable and consistent bedtimes, for weekdays and weekends.
- Most teenagers like to have a 'lie-in' at weekends – limiting the getting up time to only an hour or two later than weekdays will ensure they can get into a stable sleep routine.
- Help them to get into a routine of 30 minutes' 'quiet time' before bed – no TV, texting, homework or computer use.
- They should avoid daytime napping.
- Getting some fresh air, gentle exercise and daylight each day will help them to sleep at night.
- They should avoid caffeine and heavy exercise for 4 hours before bed, as these can cause problems getting to sleep.
- Encourage them to do their worrying before getting into bed – perhaps by writing a 'to do list' for the following day earlier in the evening.

Where can I get help?

Your GP or health visitor can offer advice and help. If things don't get better, your GP or another professional can refer your child for a specialist opinion from a paediatrician or the local child and adolescent mental health service (CAMHS). This will help to find out exactly what the problem is and how it can be best resolved.

Recommended reading

Other factsheets in this series: Worries and anxieties, CAMHS

Solve Your Child's Sleep Problems, by Dr Richard Ferber and Debbie Beckerman. A guide for parents. Published by Dorling Kindersley, 2006.

The Sleep Fairy, by Janie Peterson, Macy Peterson and Shawn Newlun. Through the story, this book teaches your child to go to sleep in their own bed to get a reward from the 'Sleep Fairy'. It has explanatory notes for parents. Published by Behave'n Kinds Press, 2003.

References

Dahl R, Harvey AG. Sleep disorders. In *Rutter's Child and Adolescent Psychiatry* (5th edn) (eds M Rutter, D Bishop, D Pine, et al): 894–905. Wiley–Blackwell, 2008.

Galland BC, Mitchell EA. Helping children sleep. *Arch Disease Childhood* 2010; 95: 850–3.

Kotagal S, Pianosi P. Sleep disorders in children and adolescents. *BMJ* 2006; 332: 828–32.

Useful websites

- **NHS Choices**: www.nhs.uk/livewell; practical hints and tips for parents.
- **Netdoctor**: www.netdoctor.co.uk; advice on sleep problems in children.
- **Mumsnet**: www.mumsnet.com; information on toddler sleep problems.

Notes

....

....

....

....

....

....

....

For a catalogue of public education materials or copies of our leaflets contact: Book Sales/Leaflets, The Royal College of Psychiatrists, 17 Belgrave Square, London SW1X 8PG. Email: leaflets@rcpsych.ac.uk, tel: 020 7235 2351 ext. 6146.

Revised by the Royal College of Psychiatrists' Child and Family Public Education Editorial Board. With grateful thanks to Dr Sarah Bates. This leaflet reflects the best possible evidence at the time of writing.

6 Behavioural problems and conduct disorder
Information for parents, carers and anyone who works with young people

This is one in a series of factsheets for parents, teachers and anyone who works with young people, with practical, up-to-date information about mental health problems (emotional, behavioural and psychiatric disorders) that can affect children and young people.

This factsheet looks at how to recognise signs of serious behavioural problems such as conduct disorder and gives some practical advice about how to deal with this and get help.

Behavioural problems – the signs

All children have moments when they do not behave properly. They can go through different phases as they develop and become more independent. Toddlers and adolescents can have their challenging moments and this might mean they push limits from time to time. With the help of parents, carers and teachers, most of them will learn to behave appropriately. Occasionally, a child will have a temper tantrum, or an outburst of aggressive or destructive behaviour, but this is often nothing to worry about.

Behavioural problems can happen in children of all ages. Some children have serious behavioural problems. The signs to look out for:

- if the child continues to behave badly for several months or longer, is repeatedly being disobedient, cheeky and aggressive
- if the child's behaviour is out of the ordinary, and seriously breaks the rules accepted in their home and school; this is much more than ordinary childish mischief or adolescent rebelliousness.

> ### What is conduct disorder?
> Sometimes, a child's behaviour can affect their development and interfere with their ability to lead a normal life. When behaviour is this much of a problem, it is called a conduct disorder.
>
> Younger children who behave disruptively and aggressively at home may be diagnosed as having 'oppositional defiant disorder'.

What does having conduct disorder mean for a young person?

Children with a conduct disorder may get involved in more violent physical fights and may steal or lie, without any sign of remorse or guilt when they are found out. They refuse to follow rules and may start to break the law. They may start to stay out all night and play truant from school during the day.

Teenagers with conduct disorder may also take risks with their health and safety by taking illegal drugs or having unprotected sexual intercourse.

What effect can this have on others?

Conduct disorder can cause a lot of distress to children, families, schools and local communities. Children who behave like this will often find it hard to make friends and have difficulties understanding social situations.

Even though they might be quite bright, they will not do well at school and are often near the bottom of the class. On the inside, the young person may be feeling that they are worthless and that they just cannot do anything right. It is common for them to show anger and to blame others for their difficulties if they do not know how to change for the better.

What causes oppositional defiant disorder/conduct disorder?

There is no single cause of conduct disorder. We are beginning to understand that there are many different possible reasons which lead to conduct disorder. A child may be more likely to develop an oppositional defiant disorder/conduct disorder if they:

- have certain genes leading to antisocial behaviour
- have difficulties learning good social and acceptable behaviours
- have a difficult temperament
- have learning or reading difficulties, making it hard for them to understand and take part in lessons; it is then easy for them to get bored, feel stupid and misbehave
- are depressed

- have been bullied or abused
- are 'hyperactive' – this causes difficulties with self-control, paying attention and following rules
- are involved with other difficult young people and drug misuse.

Other factors:

- boys are more likely to have behavioural problems and conduct disorder than girls
- parenting factors, including discipline issues and family disorganisation – parents can sometimes make things worse by giving too little attention to good behaviour, always being too quick to criticise or by being too flexible about the rules and not supervising their children.

What are the longer-term effects of conduct disorder?

A young person showing signs of conduct disorder at an early age is more likely to be male, have attention-deficit hyperactivity disorder (ADHD) and lower intelligence (general learning disability or specific difficulties in reading). The earlier the problems start, the higher the risk for the young person ending up being involved with violence and criminal acts. This may also be related to friendship groups, gangs and use of illegal substances.

What are the types of help out there?

Early diagnosis of conduct disorder and other related difficulties is important to give your child a better chance for improvement and hope for the future.

Depending on the severity of the problem, the **treatment** can be offered across different settings, for instance at home or in educational and community settings. The help offered will depend on the child's development, age and circumstances.

Involving and **supporting the family** is very important. Focusing on strengths and identifying any specific problem areas for the young person, such as learning difficulties, can improve the outcomes for young people with conduct disorders.

Help for behavioural problems can involve **supporting** the young person to increase their **positive social behaviours, and controlling** their antisocial **destructive behaviours**.

Home-based help

It can be difficult for parents and carers when their child has oppositional defiant disorder or conduct problems. You may fear your own child, and feel embarrassed or even ashamed of your child's situation. You may feel helpless and unsure how to manage it.

As a parent, it can be easy to ignore your child when they are being good and only pay attention to them when they are behaving badly. Over time, the child learns that they only get attention when they are breaking the rules. Most children, including teenagers, need a lot of attention from their parents and may be unsure how to get this. Perhaps surprisingly, they seem to prefer angry or critical attention to being ignored. It is easy to see how, over time, a vicious circle can be set up.

With children, it can help if discipline is fair and consistent and for parents/carers to agree on how to handle their child's behaviour and offer positive praise and love. This can be difficult to manage alone without the support of others, and many parents/carers require extra help.

Parenting groups can advise you on how to access the support you need, and share experiences with others who are facing similar problems with their own children. These groups can offer training in helping you encourage positive behaviour in your child.

> **Michael, 16, talks about having behavioural problems**
>
> 'My mum said that I was getting "out of control" when I was 14 years old. I was getting suspended for fighting and bunking off school. Looking back, I was not happy and I was finding schoolwork hard. I was having problems with some of the teachers at school. They said that I was causing trouble and I kept losing my temper. I was feeling really frustrated with things and getting into fights with my dad who I don't see that much.
>
> It was much better spending time with my friends. I wasn't going home when my mum wanted me there. My mum and social worker told me to go and see someone for help. I went to see someone at my local clinic who said that we all needed to have some family work to help us talk better and get me back on track. I also met with someone on my own at the clinic, and we talked about my anger and how it was affecting everyone and where it was coming from. I started thinking about ways to cope with my feelings and frustration. I still have good and bad days, but it was good to see someone who understands.' ✪

School-based help

Many young people with behavioural problems struggle at school and this can be a source of distress. School staff can help to focus on positive behaviours and reinforce work taking place at home and in the community.

Young people with behavioural problems often need help with social skills, and school may be able to offer this. Some children need individual classroom support and an assessment of learning difficulties. When the problems are severe, some children may have to be moved to special educational placements or schools where their behavioural problems can be managed.

Community-based help

If the behavioural problems are severe and persistent or a conduct disorder is suspected, ask your GP for advice.

Antisocial behaviours are commonly seen in specialist services. If specialist help is needed, the GP will make a referral to your local child and adolescent mental health service (CAMHS). This specialist team will work together with you, the school and other community groups to support you and your child.

Specialists can help to fully assess what is causing the problem and also to suggest practical ways of improving the difficult behaviour. They can also offer assessment and treatment of other conditions which can occur at the same time, such as depression, anxiety and hyperactivity.

The treatment may include social skills groups, behavioural therapy and talking therapy. These therapies can help the child to appropriately express themselves in different situations, and manage their anger more effectively.

Recommended reading

Other factsheets in this series: CAMHS, ADHD, Good parenting, General learning difficulties

National Institute for Health and Clinical Excellence. *Parent-Training/Education Programmes in the Management of Children with Conduct Disorders.* NICE, 2006.

References

Bailey S, Shooter M (eds) *The Young Mind: An Essential Guide to Mental Health for Young Adults, Parents and Teachers.* RCPsych Publications, 2009.

Rutter M, Bishop D, Pine D, et al (eds) *Rutter's Child and Adolescent Psychiatry* (5th edn). Wiley–Blackwell, 2008.

Scott S. An update on interventions for conduct disorder. *Adv Psychiatr Treat* 2008; 14: 61–70.

Useful websites

- **Samaritans**: www.samaritans.org; confidential, 24-hour emotional support to anyone in a crisis. UK helpline: 08457 909090, Irish helpline: 1850 609090, email: jo@samaritans.org.
- **Youth Justice Board**: www.justice.gov.uk/youth-justice; a public body that works to prevent offending and re-offending by children and young people under the age of 18.

Notes

7 Attention-deficit hyperactivity disorder (ADHD)
Information for parents, carers and anyone who works with young people

This is one in a series of factsheets for parents, teachers and anyone who works with young people, with practical, up-to-date information about mental health problems (emotional, behavioural and psychiatric disorders) that can affect children and young people.

This factsheet helps to understand what attention-deficit hyperactivity disorder (ADHD) is and offers some advice about what is helpful and where to get help.

How common is ADHD?

About 2 to 5% of school-age children can have ADHD. Boys are more commonly affected than girls.

What causes it?

We do not know exactly what causes this disorder, but ADHD can run in families. It is more likely in children who have significant traumatic experiences in young age. Sometimes parents feel blamed for not having controlled their child, but there is no evidence that poor parenting directly causes ADHD. However, it is important to note that parents can play a crucial role in helping and managing a child with ADHD.

What are the symptoms?

Attention-deficit hyperactivity disorder can present with different behaviours depending on the age, setting (i.e. school, home, playground) and even motivation (e.g. when doing an activity or something a child likes).

Not all children have all the symptoms. This means some can just have problems with poor attention, whereas others are mainly hyperactive.

- Children with **problems of attention** can appear forgetful, distracted, not seeming to listen, disorganised, take ages to start doing things and then when they do, they rarely finish them.
- Children with **hyperactivity** seem restless, fidgety, full of energy, 'always on the go'. They may seem loud, noisy, with a continuous chatter.
- Children with symptoms of **impulsivity** do things without thinking. They have difficulty waiting for their turn in games or in a queue, and interrupt people in conversation.

What other problems can a person with ADHD have?

Children with ADHD can have other problems such as learning difficulties, autism, conduct disorder, anxiety and depression. Neurological problems such as tics, Tourette syndrome and epilepsy can also be present. Children with ADHD can have problems with coordination or social skills and seem to be disorganised.

How long will they have ADHD?

About one in three children with a diagnosis of ADHD can grow out of their condition and not require any treatment when they are adults. The majority who receive specialist treatment tailored to their needs may

What is ADHD?

'Attention deficit disorder' (ADD), 'attention-deficit hyperactivity disorder' (ADHD), 'hyperkinetic disorder' and 'hyperactivity' are various terms used by people and professionals. These differences in terminology can sometimes cause confusion. All the above terms describe the problems of children who are hyperactive and have difficulty concentrating.

Attention-deficit hyperactivity disorder is a behavioural disorder which often becomes obvious in early childhood. The behaviours are due to underlying problems of poor attention, hyperactivity and impulsivity.

Many children, especially those under 5 years old, are inattentive and restless. This does not necessarily mean they have ADHD. The inattention or hyperactivity becomes a problem when they are exaggerated compared with other children of the same age, and when they affect the child's school, social and family life.

benefit considerably. They will have been able to catch up with their learning, improve their school performance and make friends.

Some are able to cope and manage by adapting their careers and home life. However, some can have major problems, even as adults, which may require treatment. They may also struggle with difficulties in relationships, at work, in their mood, and misuse drugs or alcohol.

How is it diagnosed?

There is no single, simple, definite test for ADHD. Making a diagnosis requires a specialist assessment, usually done by a child psychiatrist or specialist paediatrician. The diagnosis is made by recognising patterns of behaviour, observing the child, obtaining reports of their behaviour at home and at school. Sometimes a computerised test may be done to aid the diagnosis. Some children also need specialised tests by a clinical or educational psychologist.

How is it treated?

A child who has ADHD needs treatment across all situations where the difficulties occur. This means support and help at home, school, with friends and community.

It is very important for the family, teachers and other professionals to **understand** the child's condition and how it affects them. As they grow up, the young person themselves needs to be aware of their condition and how to manage it.

Teachers and parents may need to use **behavioural management strategies** such as reward charts. Parents/family may find parent training programmes helpful, especially in managing the defiant behaviours which may arise from the child's hyperactivity.

At school, children may need specific **educational support** and plans to help with their daily work in the classroom and also with homework. They may also need help to build their confidence and develop their social skills. It is important that there is good communication between home, school and the professionals treating the child to ensure that the ADHD symptoms are treated as comprehensively as possible, and that the child achieves their best potential.

Medications can play an important role in managing moderate to severe ADHD. They can help to reduce hyperactivity and improve concentration. The improved concentration gives the child the opportunity and time to learn and practise new skills. Children often say that medication helps them to get on with people, think more clearly, to understand things better and feel more in control of themselves. Not all children with ADHD will need medication.

What can I do?

A child with ADHD can present with very difficult behaviours at home, school or outside. However, there still need to be boundaries and discipline. Having ADHD does not mean the child can disobey you or behave inappropriately (e.g. swearing or being violent). A healthy lifestyle with a balanced diet and activity can help.

Children with ADHD can become easily frustrated because of their poor attention span and high energy levels. Some of the following can help manage these difficulties.

- **Give simple instructions**. Stand near them, look at them and tell them slowly and calmly what you want them to do, rather than shouting across the room.
- **Praise** your child when they have done what is required, however small it is.
- If needed, **write a list** of things to do and put it somewhere where it can be seen clearly (e.g. door of their room, bathroom).
- Break any task, like doing homework or sitting by the dining table, to **smaller time spans** (15–20 min).
- Give them **time and activities** to spend their energy on, for example playing football or swimming.

> **Ben, 11**
>
> 'I was always getting into trouble at school. The teacher used to tell me off for not sitting still. I'd try to sit down but it was hard – I would just want to get up and walk around. I was always getting into trouble for talking. The other children in my class could sit and finish their work, but I found this hard.
>
> Mum and Dad said I had a lot of energy. Sometimes my friends would tell me I was over the top. Mum says she couldn't take me anywhere when I was younger because I was so noisy and always on the go.
>
> In the end, Mum and Dad took me to a clinic for children who have problems. They said I have ADHD and talked to my parents and teachers about how to help me. They gave me some medication which I take every day. Everyone thinks it helps. I don't seem to get told off so much and I can sit and do my schoolwork now.' ✪

- Change their **diet** and avoid additives. There is some evidence about the effect of diet on some children; they may be sensitive to certain food additives and colourings. If parents notice that certain foods worsen the child's hyperactivity, these should be avoided. It is best to discuss this with your doctor or specialist dietitian.
- Many parents find it helpful to attend **parenting programmes**, irrespective of whether the child is being treated for ADHD. Some areas offer parenting programmes and support groups specifically for parents of children with ADHD.

How do I get help?

The child's GP, teacher or school nurse can refer them to a specialist (e.g. a paediatrician or a child and adolescent mental health service – CAMHS). The specialist will complete an assessment and offer treatment.

Additional information on medications for ADHD

Medications used to treat ADHD are broadly divided into two groups:
- stimulants such as methylphenidate and dexamphetamine
- non-stimulants such as atomoxetine.

Stimulants

Stimulants have the effect of making people feel more alert, energetic and awake. In a person with ADHD, they can improve attention and reduce hyperactivity. The stimulants used in the treatment of ADHD include methylphenidate (previously commonly known by the name 'ritalin') and dexamphetamine.

Methylphenidate is available in different forms. Immediate-release methylphenidate is short acting. It is used for its flexibility in dosing and can be used to determine the correct level of dose during dose changes. Slow- or modified-release methylphenidate works for 8–12 hours and can be given once a day. This is more convenient, and as the child or young person need not take a dose in school, reduces the stigma attached to ADHD.

Non-stimulants

Non-stimulant medications by nature do not make people alert or active. However, in ADHD, they can improve symptoms of inattention and hyperactivity. These include medications like atomoxetine.

Other drugs

Sometimes other medications may be used to help with problems with sleep and challenging behaviours that are associated with ADHD.

How do they work?

Medications act on certain chemicals in the brain called noradrenaline. They seem to affect the parts of the brain that control attention and organise our behaviour. They do not cure ADHD, but they help to control the symptoms of poor attention, overactivity or impulsivity.

Which medication will be used for my child?

Stimulant medication methylphenidate is usually prescribed first. The type of stimulant prescribed will depend on a number of things such as the symptoms your child has, your choice of treatment, the ease of giving the medication and even its availability and cost.

If methylphenidate causes unpleasant side-effects or does not work, other stimulant (dexamphetamine) or non-stimulant medications may be prescribed. Sometimes a child may respond to a different form of methylphenidate.

How do I know it is working?

You will find that:
- your child's concentration is better
- their feelings of restlessness or overactivity are less
- they control themselves better.

Sometimes school or teachers notice the improvement before you do.

What are the side-effects?

As with most medications, there may be some unwanted effects. However, not everyone gets side-effects and most are mild and disappear with continued use. Side-effects are less likely if the dose is increased gradually when the tablets are started. Some parents worry about addiction, but there is no good evidence to suggest that this is a problem.

Some of the common side-effects of methylphenidate:

- loss of appetite
- difficulty falling asleep
- light-headedness.

Less common side-effects to look out for include:

- being 'overfocused', quiet and staring – this may be a sign that the dose is too high
- anxiety, nervousness, irritability or tearfulness
- tummy pains or feeling sick
- headache, dizziness or drowsiness
- tics or twitches.

In the long term, sometimes growth slows down when children are on methylphenidate. Research shows that the total adult height may be reduced by 2.5 cm when taking methylphenidate as a child.

This list of side-effects is not exhaustive. **If you notice anything unusual, it is important to contact your doctor immediately.**

Is there anything I need to know before giving the medication?

Before you give any medication tell your doctor about:

- allergies your child might have
- any other medicines they take, including vitamins or supplements
- for older girls, if they are likely to become pregnant
- if you or anyone in your family has physical health problems, especially high blood pressure, heart problems and repeated movements (tics).

Are there any special tests before or while taking the medication?

Before taking the medication, your child should have a physical check-up, especially for their heart rate, blood pressure, growth and any other medical problems. Sometimes they may need a blood test or heart tracing test to measure the electrical activity of the heart. This is called an electrocardiogram (ECG).

While taking the medication, the doctor will monitor your child's heart rate, blood pressure, weight and height on a regular basis along with checking for any side-effects.

What do I need to know about giving the medication?

Do

- Give the medication at the times you were told by the doctor or pharmacist.
- Keep appointments for regular review of medication.
- Store the medication safely.
- Ensure your child swallows the medication, not chews or crushes it.
- Make sure your child drinks enough, especially in hot weather and while exercising.

Don't

- Double the dose if they miss a dose of medication.
- Stop giving the medication without discussing this with the doctor.
- Give the medication to anyone else, even if you feel their difficulties are similar to your child's.

How long do they need to be on the medication?

Most children and young people need the medication at least until they finish their education or schooling. A few might need to take it even when they grow up. Some children need medications only at specific times, for example while attending school, and do not have to take it on weekends or on school holidays. Your doctor would regularly check, at least once a year, if they need to continue the medicine.

Taking these medications can affect driving and even certain careers, such as joining the army. It is important that the child is aware of this and will need to discuss it with their doctor as they grow up.

Young people may need explanations and support as they grow up about taking their medication. Stopping medication can cause symptoms to return, and some young people can put themselves at risk in terms of their education, their work, and socially by being impulsive and taking alcohol or drugs.

Remember: if you have any further questions regarding psychiatric medication, do not hesitate to contact your doctor or pharmacist.

Recommended reading

Other factsheets in this series:
Restless and excitable child, CAMHS

Recommended for parents/professionals

ADD/ADHD Behavior Change Resource Kit: Ready-to-Use Strategies & Activities for Helping Children with Attention Deficit Disorder, by Grad L. Flick. A useful book published by Jossey Bass, 1998.

The AD/HD Handbook: A Guide for Parents and Professionals on Attention Deficit/Hyperactivity Disorder, written by Dr Alison Munden and Dr Jon Arcelus. Jessica Kingsley Publishers, 1999.

Recommended for children

Everything a Child Needs to Know about ADHD, for children aged 6–12 years. Written by Dr C. R. Yemula, ADDISS, 2007.

Putting on the Brakes: Young People's Guide to Understanding Attention Deficit Hyperactivity Disorder, for ages 8–12. Written by Dr Patricia O. Quinn and Dr Judith M. Stern, American Psychological Association, 2001.

References

British National Formulary, 62th Edition (September 2011) British Medical Association and Royal Pharmaceutical Society of Great Britain, 2011.

National Institute for Health and Clinical Excellence. *Attention Deficit Hyperactivity Disorder: Diagnosis and Management of ADHD in Children, Young People and Adults* (CG72). NICE, 2008.

National Institute for Health and Clinical Excellence. *Methylphenidate, Atomoxetine and Dexamfetamine for the Treatment of Attention Deficit Hyperactivity Disorder in Children and Adolescents (review)* (TA98). NICE, 2006.

Pelsser LM, Frankena K, Toorman J, et al. Effects of a restricted elimination diet on the behaviour of children with attention-deficit hyperactivity disorder (INCA study): a randomised controlled trial. *Lancet* 2011; 377: 494–503.

Rutter M, Bishop D, Pine D, et al (eds) *Rutter's Child and Adolescent Psychiatry* (5th edn). Wiley–Blackwell, 2008.

Useful websites

- **ADD Information and Support Services (ADDISS)**: www.addiss.co.uk; information and resources about ADHD to anyone who needs assistance.

- **Young Minds**: www.youngminds.org.uk; information and helpline for any adult concerned about the emotions and behaviour of a child or young person. Parents' helpline: 0808 802 5544.

- **ADD Resources**: www.addresources.org; free and carefully chosen articles helpful to adults with ADD/ADHD and to parents of children with ADD/ADHD, links to other ADHD-related websites, and more.

- **Electronic Medicines Compendium (eMC)**: www.medicines.org.uk; information about UK-licensed medicines.

Notes

8 The child with general learning disability
Information for parents, carers and anyone who works with young people

This is one in a series of factsheets for parents, teachers and anyone who works with young people, with practical, up-to-date information about mental health problems (emotional, behavioural and psychiatric disorders) that can affect children and young people.

This factsheet describes what a general learning disability is and what the possible causes may be. It also provides practical advice about the help that is available to young people with a general learning disability and their family.

What causes general learning disability?

In many children with general learning disability the cause of the disability remains unknown. In some there may be genetic factors, infection, brain injury or damage before birth, at birth or after. Examples include Down syndrome, fragile-X syndrome and cerebral palsy.

The effects of learning disability

Children or young people who have a general learning disability are aware of what goes on around them. However, their ability to understand and communicate may be limited, and they can find it hard to express themselves. Speech problems can make it even harder to make other people understand their feelings and needs.

They can become frustrated and upset by their own limitations. When they compare themselves with other children, they can feel sad or angry and think badly of themselves.

For a parent, it can be distressing to find out that their child has a general learning disability. It may be hard for them and other members of the family to understand why the child is like this. It can also be hard to communicate with the child, difficult to manage their behaviour and hard for other people to understand.

Brothers and sisters may be affected in a number of ways. They may feel jealous of the attention given to their brother or sister who has a disability, or they may be embarrassed by their behaviour. They may even be teased at school. Quite often, they can feel personally responsible for their disabled sibling or their distressed parent.

Learning disability and mental health

A general learning disability is not a mental illness. However, children with learning disability are more likely than other children to develop mental health problems, for example anxiety, or have additional developmental disorders, such as an autism spectrum disorder or attention-deficit hyperactivity disorder (ADHD).

What can be done to help?

Recognising difficulties in learning and development

It is important to recognise as soon as possible that a child is learning and developing slowly. It is only when the problem is recognised that the child and their family can be offered the help and support they need. The **health visitor** plays an important role in identifying slow development in the years before school.

What is meant by learning disability?

Learning disability used to be known as mental handicap or mental retardation. Other terms sometimes used are 'general' or 'global developmental delay' and 'intellectual disability'.

A child with a general learning disability finds it more difficult to learn, understand and do things compared with other children of the same age. Like all children and young people, children with learning disabilities can continue to progress and learn throughout their childhood, but more slowly.

The degree of disability can vary greatly. Some children with severe disability will never learn to speak and when they grow up, will need help with looking after themselves: feeding, dressing or going to the toilet. Other children with mild learning disability can grow up to be independent.

'General learning disability' is different from 'specific learning difficulty' which means that the person has difficulties in one or two areas of their learning, but manages well in other areas of their development. For example, a child can have a specific learning difficulty in reading, writing or understanding what is said to them, but have no problem with learning skills in other areas of life.

Beth, 15, who has a moderate learning disability

'Beth was referred to us by her paediatrician who was concerned for her mental health. She had deliberately swallowed two antacid tablets and two diet pills. She had been increasingly aggressive and restless both at home and school. She was barely sleeping at night, was "talking gibberish" and very fast, running away and taking her clothes off inappropriately.

There had been similar episodes in the past for varying periods, but none had been this severe. There was family history of schizophrenia and bipolar disorder. Beth was diagnosed with bipolar affective disorder. She was prescribed medication – a mood stabiliser – and her state improved. A year later, Beth started becoming more agitated, and tearful. She had developed an episode of depression and needed an antidepressant. She has now recovered to her previous self. Beth is likely to have high and low episodes like these, especially if not on treatment. She will need to be monitored for a long time.

People with learning disability can have major mental illness like others. The way they appear to professionals will be different and they will need to see specialists who will look at behaviour and recognise any patterns suggestive of a psychiatric disorder.' ✪

Child development team

As the child gets older, a number of people can help with their particular needs. They will often work together in a group known as the 'child development team'. This team comprises specialists such as community paediatricians, nurses, psychologists and speech therapists. It sometimes includes a child psychiatrist or other members of the child and adolescent mental health service (CAMHS). In some areas, there are special services for children with learning disabilities (community learning disability team). If necessary, a GP can refer the child to one of these specialist teams.

Schooling

School can be a particular challenge for children with learning disabilities because of both the learning and social demands. Local education departments can make special arrangements to meet the educational needs of each child. Usually there is an expectation that most children will receive their education in a mainstream inclusive environment. For example, children who are able to cope comfortably with other people are likely to attend an ordinary school, but have **special** forms of **teaching**. On the other hand, a child with a more severe disability may go to a **special school**.

For some children, an educational psychologist will prepare a **Statement of Special Educational Needs**. This sets out what special help the child needs, and takes into account the views and wishes of the child and their parents.

All educational authorities have a **Parent Partnership Scheme** (www.parentpartnership.org.uk) to advise parents on educational provision.

In most areas, there are also other services. **Respite care** and **holiday play schemes** can extend the learning and social opportunities for the child. **Parent support groups** can put families in touch with other people who are coping with similar problems. The local Social Services department will be able to advise, both on these opportunities and on the **benefits** to which parents are entitled.

Disability does not stop a child from having a full and enjoyable life. The aim of all the specialist services is to help children with a general learning disability and their families to have lives that are as enjoyable and fulfilling as those of other people.

Notes

Recommended reading

Other factsheets in this series:
Specific learning difficulties, CAMHS

Books Beyond Words: www.booksbeyondwords.co.uk; a series of picture books for use by people with learning disabilities to make communication easier and allow for discussion.

First Impressions, a booklet about emotional and practical support for families of young children with learning disabilities. Published by the Foundation for People with Learning Disabilities.

Information for people with learning disability and their carers: The Royal College of Psychiatrists' Faculty of the Psychiatry of Intellectual Disability and the Leicestershire Partnership NHS Trust have produced accessible information for people with mental health problems and learning disabilities. All these materials have been written and tested with people with learning disabilities and their carers (www.rcpsych.ac.uk/mentalhealthinfo/problems/learningdisabilities.aspx).

Mental Health Needs of Children and Young People with Learning Disabilities, edited by R. Raghavan, S. Bernard and J. McCarthy. Pavilion Press, 2010.

Seeing the Psychologist for a Cognitive Assessment: a leaflet by Cheshire and Wirral Partnership NHS Foundation Trust, available here: www.cwp.nhs.uk/Publications/Leaflets/ldleaflets/Pages/Assessments.aspx.

The Young Mind: An Essential Guide to Mental Health for Young Adults, Parents and Teachers, edited by Sue Bailey and Mike Shooter (2009) – an accessible, user-friendly handbook produced by the Royal College of Psychiatrists.

References

Bernard S, Turk J (eds) *Developing Mental Health Services for Children and Adolescents with Learning Disabilities: A Toolkit for Clinicians*. RCPsych Publications, 2009.

Gillberg C, Harrington R, Steinhausen H-C (eds) *A Clinician's Handbook of Child and Adolescent Psychiatry* (1st edn). Cambridge University Press, 2006.

Rutter M, Bishop D, Pine D, et al (eds) *Rutter's Child and Adolescent Psychiatry* (5th edn). Wiley–Blackwell, 2008.

Useful websites

⊃ **Contact a Family**: www.cafamily.org.uk; information and advice for parents of children with any special needs or disability.

⊃ **MENCAP**: www.mencap.org.uk; leading UK charity for people with learning disabilities.

⊃ **Every Disabled Child Matters**: www.edcm.org.uk; campaign to get rights and justice for every child with a disability.

⊃ **UK Government website for citizens**: www.direct.gov.uk; useful information regarding special educational needs and navigating through the Statement of Special Educational Needs process.

⊃ **Disability and Inclusion**: www.barnardos.org.uk; Barnardo's is committed to the principle of inclusion for disabled children and works with children from pre-school age to 16+.

⊃ **The Children's Trust**: www.thechildrenstrust.org.uk; national charity working with children who have multiple disabilities.

⊃ **British Institute of Learning Disabilities**: www.bild.org.uk; useful information to support people with learning disabilities and their families.

⊃ **The Royal College of Psychiatrists' Faculty of the Psychiatry of Intellectual Disability and the Leicestershire Partnership NHS Trust**: www.rcpsych.ac.uk/mentalhealthinfo/problems/learningdisabilities.aspx; accessible information for people with mental health problems and learning disabilities which has been written and tested with people with learning disabilities and their carers.

For a catalogue of public education materials or copies of our leaflets contact: Book Sales/Leaflets, The Royal College of Psychiatrists, 17 Belgrave Square, London SW1X 8PG. Email: leaflets@rcpsych.ac.uk, tel: 020 7235 2351 ext. 6146.

Revised by the Royal College of Psychiatrists' Child and Family Public Education Editorial Board. With grateful thanks to Lakshmiprabha Ramasubramanian, Alison Dunkerley and Krishna Madhusudhan. This leaflet reflects the best possible evidence at the time of writing.

9 Specific learning difficulties
Information for parents, carers and anyone who works with young people

This is one in a series of factsheets for parents, teachers and anyone who works with young people, with practical, up-to-date information about mental health problems (emotional, behavioural and psychiatric disorders) that can affect children and young people.

This factsheet explores what a specific learning difficulty is and gives advice on where and how to get help for young people affected by this condition and for their families.

What effect does it have?

Specific learning difficulties can make lessons challenging for a child. They may struggle keeping up with classmates, and may come to see themselves as stupid or no good.

If the child finds it difficult to concentrate on lessons, because they may not be able to follow them properly, they may complain of lessons being 'boring' and search for other ways to pass the time and to succeed.

They may try to avoid doing schoolwork because they find it impossible to do it well. Doing badly in school can undermine their self-confidence, and this can make it harder for them to get along with other children and to keep friends.

Children with specific reading difficulties often become angry and frustrated, so behavioural problems are common. If they don't get suitable help, the problems may get worse. Older children may become frustrated, fail exams or get into serious trouble, both at school and outside.

A specific learning difficulty is not a mental illness. However, children with a specific learning difficulty are more likely than other children to develop mental health problems, for example anxiety, or have additional developmental disorders, such as autism spectrum disorder and attention-deficit hyperactivity disorder (ADHD).

What can help?

Identifying the problem is the most important step to get the right help and support. Usually the difficulties are first picked up by the family or school.

Parents can discuss their concerns with the teacher or special educational needs coordinating officer (SENCO). Education authorities have a **duty** to identify children who have special educational needs and make sure that they get the **additional help** that they require (Education Act 1990). Schools have the *Special Educational Needs Code of Practice*, drawn up by the Department for Education, to help them to recognise and assist children with this type of problem. The Department for Education has also produced a guide for parents and carers.

If there are concerns, the school may offer extra help using different ways of teaching to suit the child's specific needs (called **individual education plan** or IEP). If this is not enough, then they can offer interventions that are additional to, or different from, those provided as part of the school's usual curriculum and strategies (School Action and School Action Plus).

Sometimes a statutory assessment may be required for the education authority to prepare a **Statement of Special Educational Needs**. This would describe what type of additional help the child will benefit from, and is usually reviewed annually.

Children may need to see an educational psychologist, speech and language therapist or other specialist to diagnose their problem.

What is a specific learning difficulty?

When talking about 'specific learning difficulties', it is more common to apply the term 'difficulty' rather than 'disability' which is used in people affected with more general disability, although these labels are used differently in different settings such as healthcare, education and government.

A child with a 'specific learning difficulty' is as able as any other child, except in one or two areas of their learning. For instance, they may find it difficult to write letters (dysgraphia), or to cope with numbers (dyscalculia) or reading (dyslexia).

There are many different types of specific learning difficulties, but the best known is probably dyslexia. In dyslexia, the child finds it hard to spell and read. It may be difficult for parents and teachers to realise that a child has this sort of problem, especially if their development has progressed without concern in the early years.

Often, the child will appear to understand, have good ideas, and join in storytelling and other activities as well as other children, and better than some. Sometimes it can take years for adults to realise that a child has a specific learning difficulty.

If the child's learning problem has resulted in possible emotional or behaviour problems, owing to frustration or loss of self-confidence, more specialist help may be needed. If necessary, the school or GP can refer the child to the local child and adolescent mental health service (CAMHS) who will be able to offer help and support.

Recommended reading

Other factsheets in this series:
Autism, ADHD, CAMHS

The Young Mind: An Essential Guide to Mental Health for Young Adults, Parents and Teachers, edited by Sue Bailey and Mike Shooter (2009) – an accessible, user-friendly handbook produced by the Royal College of Psychiatrists.

Special Educational Needs (SEN) – A Guide for Parents and Carers (revised 2009), published by the UK Department for Children, Schools and Families. It is free to download (https://www.education.gov.uk/publications/standard/Healthanddisabilities/Page1/DCSF-00639-2008).

References

Gillberg C, Harrington R, Steinhausen H-C (eds) *A Clinician's Handbook of Child and Adolescent Psychiatry* (1st edn). Cambridge University Press, 2006.

Rutter M, Bishop D, Pine D, et al (eds) *Rutter's Child and Adolescent Psychiatry* (5th edn). Wiley–Blackwell, 2008.

Useful websites

- **Advisory Centre for Education**: www.ace-ed.org.uk; national charity that provides advice and information to parents and carers on a wide range of school-related issues including exclusion, admissions, special educational needs, bullying and attendance.

- **Department for Education**: www.education.gov.uk/childrenandyoungpeople/send; information for parents and carers on special educational needs, a helpful guide to the process and some useful addresses.

- **British Dyslexia Association**: www.bdadyslexia.org.uk; information and advice on dyslexia for people with dyslexia and those who support them. Helpline: 0845 251 9002.

- **Independent Parental Special Educational Advice**: www.ipsea.org.uk; information and second opinions for special educational needs.

- **Young Minds**: www.youngminds.org.uk; for any adult concerned about the emotions and behaviour of a child or young person. Parents' helpline: 0808 802 5544.

- **UK Government website for citizens**: www.direct.gov.uk; useful information regarding special educational needs and navigating through the statement process.

- **The Royal College of Psychiatrists' Faculty of the Psychiatry of Intellectual Disability and the Leicestershire Partnership NHS Trust**: www.rcpsych.ac.uk/mentalhealthinfo/problems/learningdisabilities.aspx; accessible information for people with mental health problems and intellectual disabilities which has been written and tested with people with intellectual disabilities and their carers.

Daniel, 12, talks about his dyslexia

'When I was 6, I had trouble learning the alphabet and could not spell words. I couldn't concentrate and always found excuses not do my schoolwork. My friends thought I was lazy and stupid. I was too shy to tell my teacher that I couldn't do my work; I thought I was just thick.

My parents would get upset with me when I couldn't do my schoolwork or read my school books as they wanted me to keep up with my friends. I had a hard time at school and was too embarrassed to ask for help.

Then, when I was 7, my teacher told my parents that I could have dyslexia because I could not read properly and my handwriting was messy and jumbled. I had some tests and then they told me that I had dyslexia. Suddenly, I felt like they understood me and I was not a lazy boy after all.

The school has now provided me with a lot of help and has made so many changes for me so that I can learn and achieve. Now I use a word processor with grammar and a spell checker quite well and I am pleased to say that I am doing so much better. I have made friends and my confidence has improved a lot.' ✪

Notes

....

....

....

....

....

....

....

For a catalogue of public education materials or copies of our leaflets contact: Book Sales/Leaflets, The Royal College of Psychiatrists, 17 Belgrave Square, London SW1X 8PG. Email: leaflets@rcpsych.ac.uk, tel: 020 7235 2351 ext. 6146.

Revised by the Royal College of Psychiatrists' Child and Family Public Education Editorial Board. With grateful thanks to Lakshmiprabha Ramasubramanian. This leaflet reflects the best possible evidence at the time of writing.
The Royal College of Psychiatrists is a charity registered in England and Wales (228636) and in Scotland (SC038369). © The Royal College of Psychiatrists 2013

10 Autism and Asperger syndrome
Information for parents, carers and anyone who works with young people

This is one in a series of factsheets for parents, teachers and anyone who works with young people, with practical, up-to-date information about mental health problems (emotional, behavioural and psychiatric disorders) that can affect children and young people.

This factsheet gives details about autism spectrum disorder and offers practical advice about how to get help if you think your child has such a disorder.

What does autism spectrum disorder mean?

Children and young people with autism spectrum disorder have articular difficulties:

- in communicating
- being around people socially, and
- with their behaviour.

Individuals with an autism spectrum disorder can have a range of intellectual ability from having severe intellectual disabilities, to being more academically able and in mainstream education. About 10% of people with autism may also have some special skills and abilities.

For a diagnosis of autism, there must be evidence of unusual development in the first three years of life. 'Asperger syndrome' is a term used for some higher-functioning people on the autism spectrum who have intellectual ability in the average range and no delays in learning to talk. Many often have intense interests such as train timetables, buses or dinosaurs.

What are the characteristics?

The characteristics of children and young people with autism spectrum disorder will vary depending on their age, developmental level and how severely they are affected.

The difficulties are also likely to change over time. Parents are usually (but not always) the first to have some concerns about their child's development, and difficulties may be noticed from as early as infancy.

Overall, the problems and behaviours can be divided into three main areas.

- **Difficulties with communication**

  Children and young people with autism spectrum disorder have difficulties with both verbal communication (speaking) and non-verbal communication (eye contact, expressions and gestures). Some children may not be able to talk at all or have very limited speech.

  Some have good speech and language skills, but still have difficulty using their speech socially or to maintain a conversation. Their use of language may be very formal or 'adult-like'. They may talk at length about their own topics of interest, but find it hard to understand the back-and-forth nature of two-way conversations.

- **Difficulties with social interaction**

  Children and young people with autism spectrum disorder have difficulty understanding the 'social world', for example, they often struggle with recognising and understanding their own feelings and those of people around them. This in turn can make it difficult for them to make friends. They may prefer to spend time alone, or appear insensitive to others because of their difficulties understanding social rules and expectations. Others may want to make friends, but have difficulties understanding someone else's point of view.

- **Difficulties with behaviour, interests and activities**

  Children and young people with autism spectrum disorder often prefer familiar routines (e.g. taking the same route to school every day, putting their clothes on in a particular order), and tend to find it hard to deal with change, which they find upsetting.

What are autism spectrum disorders?

Autism is the central condition in the group of disorders known as 'autism spectrum disorders' or 'autism spectrum conditions'. They have also been called 'social and communication disorders' or 'pervasive developmental disorders'. For simplicity, we will use the term autism spectrum disorders.

These are neurodevelopmental disorders, which means they are caused by abnormalities in the way the brain develops and works.

Autism spectrum disorders affect approximately 1 in 100 children and young people.

They may also have unusual intense and specific interests, such as in electronic gadgets or lists of dates. They might use toys more like 'objects' to line up, for example. They may also have unusual responses to particular experiences from their environment, such as tastes, smells, sounds and textures. For example, they could be very sensitive to the sound of a hair dryer or the feel of certain materials against their skin.

Some children show unusual repetitive movements, such as hand or finger flapping or twisting, or complicated whole-body movements.

What are the causes?

The exact cause of autism spectrum disorder is unknown, although research shows that a combination of genetic and environmental factors may account for changes in brain development. There is an increased risk of autism spectrum disorder and other developmental difficulties in the brothers and sisters of children with autism spectrum disorder.

Where can I get help?

If you are worried about your child's development, or their school or nursery has contacted you about their worries, the first step is to speak to your GP or health visitor. They will advise you, and make a referral, if necessary, to the local autism spectrum disorder diagnostic team at the child development team or child and adolescent mental health service (CAMHS).

Making the correct diagnosis requires a detailed discussion about your child's early development, a medical and psychological assessment, and a comprehensive assessment of your child's social and communication skills and intellectual abilities. Some of this will be done by watching your child in different settings, for example at school. There is no single test (e.g. blood test or brain scan) for autism spectrum disorder, but several different tests (e.g. hearing tests and blood tests) may be carried out to exclude other conditions.

> **Kester, 9**
>
> 'I like playing on my computer and role-playing games. It's OK playing on the computer because I can find people who like the same things as me. Most of the kids at school think I am weird when I talk to them about my games. My mum worries that I want to stay in my room and not see other kids my age after school. I prefer to be on my own – other kids wind me up and then I lose my temper. As I get older, I hope to make friends with other people who enjoy the same things as me.
>
> My mum says I have got Asperger syndrome. I don't really understand what this is but I don't care. I know it means I am different from other kids – that I find it difficult to get on with other kids. My mum doesn't always understand when I want to do things like not wanting to wear socks or shoes. I do wear them to school but I take them off as soon as I get home.' ✪

Learning difficulties

Children with autism spectrum disorder can have general or specific learning disabilities which may range from mild to severe. Like all children, they will have their own strengths and difficulties, both with their learning and their abilities.

What can be done to help?

There are no known cures for autism spectrum disorder, but children and families can be helped in many ways, for example, by:

- being given information about the condition
- managing behavioural difficulties
- developing social communication and emotional skills
- in some cases, medication.

There are various approaches available to help with communication and learning, and it is often better to get help as early as possible. Usually, there will be several people involved in the care of a child with autism spectrum disorder – a speech and language therapist, psychologist, occupational therapist and a medical doctor (paediatrician or child psychiatrist).

There might also be specialist courses on parenting, parent support groups, advice on how to help the wider family and more general advice about benefits, for example, from local child health services and independent organisations such as the National Autistic Society.

Education

Children and young people with autism spectrum disorder often need special educational support. This may be in a special school, or in a mainstream school with extra help to manage conflict and upset feelings and help them to get on with other people for example. Unstructured situations, such as break and lunch times, can be very difficult for some children with autism spectrum disorder who may be vulnerable to bullying or exploitation, particularly in secondary schools.

The future

Most children and young people with autism spectrum disorder continue to experience similar difficulties throughout life, although generally they become less severe over time. Getting help as early as possible for children and young people with autism spectrum disorder can make a real difference.

Additional resources

Social Services can have a role to play in providing practical support and help for the young person and their family – accessing local services and resources, such as respite care, and advice on disability allowances. Many families also value support from their local autism parent and carer support group.

Recommended reading

Other factsheets in this series: General learning disability, Specific learning difficulties, CAMHS

Finding Out About Asperger's Syndrome, High-Functioning Autism and PDD, by Gunilla Gerland. Jessica Kingsley Publishers, 2000.

It Can Get Better: Dealing with Common Behaviour Problems in Young Autistic Children. A Guide for Parents and Carers, by Paul Dickinson and Liz Hannah. Central, 1998.

Parenting a Child with Asperger Syndrome: 200 Tips and Strategies, by B. Boyd. Jessica Kingsley Publishers, 2003.

The ASD Workbook: Understanding your Autism Spectrum Disorder, by Penny Kershaw. Jessica Kingsley Publishers, 2011.

The Complete Guide to Asperger's Syndrome, by Tony Attwood. Jessica Kingsley Publishers, 2006.

The Young Mind: An Essential Guide to Mental Health for Young Adults, Parents and Teachers, edited by Sue Bailey and Mike Shooter (2009) – an accessible, user-friendly handbook produced by the Royal College of Psychiatrists.

References

National Institute for Health and Clinical Excellence. *Autism: Recognition, Referral and Diagnosis of Children and Young People on the Autism Spectrum* (CG128). NICE, 2011.

Rutter M, Bishop D, Pine D, et al (eds) *Rutter's Child and Adolescent Psychiatry* (5th edn). Wiley–Blackwell, 2008.

Scottish Intercollegiate Guidelines Network. *Assessment, Diagnosis and Clinical Interventions for Children and Young People with Autism Spectrum Disorders: A National Clinical Guideline* (CG98). SIGN, 2007.

Scottish Intercollegiate Guidelines Network. *Autism Spectrum Disorders: Booklet for Young People*. SIGN, 2009.

Useful websites

⊃ **The National Autistic Society**: www.autism.org.uk; champions the rights and interests of all people with autism and aims to provide individuals with autism and their families with help, support and accessible services.

⊃ **Contact a Family**: www.cafamily.org.uk; UK-wide charity providing advice, information and support to parents of children with a disability. Helpline: 0808 808 3555.

⊃ **Research Autism**: www.researchautism.net; a UK charity dedicated to research into interventions in autism.

⊃ **The Royal College of Psychiatrists' Faculty of the Psychiatry of Intellectual Disability and the Leicestershire Partnership NHS Trust**: www.rcpsych.ac.uk/mentalhealthinfo/problems/ learningdisabilities.aspx; accessible information for people with mental health problems and intellectual disabilities which has been written and tested with people with intellectual disabilities and their carers.

For a catalogue of public education materials or copies of our leaflets contact: Book Sales/Leaflets, The Royal College of Psychiatrists, 17 Belgrave Square, London SW1X 8PG. Email: leaflets@rcpsych.ac.uk, tel: 020 7235 2351 ext. 6146.

Revised by the Royal College of Psychiatrists' Child and Family Public Education Editorial Board. With grateful thanks to Dr Professor Ann Le Couteur. This leaflet reflects the best possible evidence at the time of writing.

11 Depression in children
Information for parents, carers and anyone who works with young people

This is one in a series of factsheets for parents, teachers and anyone who works with young people, with practical, up-to-date information about mental health problems (emotional, behavioural and psychiatric disorders) that can affect children and young people.

This factsheet gives some basic information about the symptoms and effects of depression in children and adolescents, and gives practical advice on how to get help for this problem.

How common is depression?

Depression is thought to occur in around 1–3% of children and young people.

Anybody can have depression and it happens in people of all ages, races, income levels and educational levels. Teenage girls are twice as likely as teenage boys to be depressed.

What causes depression?

There is no specific cause for depression. It can be caused by a mixture of things, rather than any one thing alone. It may be triggered by stressful life events, for example bullying at school, parental separation or divorce, bereavement or conflicts with family members or friends. It can also run in families, especially if a parent has depression or a mood disorder such as bipolar disorder (also called 'manic depression').

> ### What is depression?
> Feeling sad or fed up is a normal reaction to experiences that are difficult or stressful. Sometimes these feelings of sadness can go on for some time and can start to interfere with everyday life. At these times the low moods become part of an illness we call 'depression'.

What are the symptoms of depression?

When a child or young person is depressed many changes can be seen. They may:

- lose interest in activities that they enjoyed before
- lose their appetite or start overeating
- have problems with concentration, remembering things or making decisions
- self-harm or have thoughts of suicide
- have disturbed sleep or sleep far too much
- feel tired all the time, exhausted
- complain of aches and pains, for example headaches or tummy pains
- have little self-confidence
- express feelings of guilt for no reason.

In children, especially teenagers, being irritable and grumpy all the time can also be a symptom of depression, not just of being in a 'bad mood'.

At the extreme end of depression, some young people can develop 'psychotic symptoms' – they may start to have very unusual and sometimes unpleasant thoughts and experiences.

Some children also have periods of high mood (also called 'mania') along with periods of low mood. This may mean they have bipolar mood disorder.

What effects can depression have on the young person?

A child or young person with depression can have major problems in not only how they feel, but also how they behave. This may cause difficulties at home, at school, as well as with relationships with family and friends. Some young people may try to cope with their problems by engaging in risky behaviours, such as self-harming (e.g. cutting), misusing drugs or alcohol, having inappropriate sexual relationships (leading to teen pregnancy in girls), dropping out of school, and, at the extreme end, suicide.

The longer the illness continues without understanding, help or treatment, the more harmful it is likely to be to the life of the young person and to their family.

Angela talks about her 16-year-old daughter's depression

'Millie was 15 when she started staying up late at night, not sleeping, eating a lot and spending most of the time in her room. We thought this was because the demands from school had increased. We didn't even really notice that she wasn't meeting up her friends or talking to us like usual. We took her to see the doctor because we thought she was a bit down and pale. The doctor was concerned and asked her questions which opened our eyes.

I soon noticed that Millie had started cutting herself. When I confronted her about this she became upset – she accused us of "having a go". She said she just couldn't be bothered anymore with anything .The more we talked, the more Millie started to acknowledge that she needed help. She told us she couldn't enjoy things anymore like she used to. She couldn't focus on her schoolwork and was falling behind. Teachers were noticing this, saying she wasn't getting on with her work.

We took Millie back to her doctor and then to see a therapist at CAMHS. It wasn't until Millie started to talk about how she was feeling that things started to change. We are just so pleased the help was there when Millie needed it. Now, Millie has moved further on and will soon be starting college. She is now back to her usual self.' ✪

Where can I get help?

Depression is a treatable illness. The first step towards getting help is to recognise that there might be a problem. It might help to talk to others who know your child. For instance, contact the school to find how they are doing.

If you suspect that a young person is depressed, seeking medical advice early on is very important. As a first step, you should contact your GP. If necessary, they can then make a referral to your local child and adolescent mental health service (CAMHS) which can offer more specialist help.

How is depression treated?

The goal of treatment is to improve the symptoms, prevent the illness from returning and help the young person lead a normal life. Families play an important role in recognising the illness, supporting the young person through treatment and also preventing the illness from coming back. It is therefore very important that you understand the condition.

Depending on how depression is affecting your child and how severe it is, they may need different treatments. When they have severe symptoms or have difficulties such as serious suicidal thoughts or other risky behaviours, they may need medication and sometimes admission to hospital.

Psychological ('talking') treatments and medication both may have an important role in the treatment of depression.

Talking treatments (also known as 'psychotherapies')

Psychological therapies such as cognitive–behavioural therapy (CBT) or 'interpersonal therapy' may be tried before considering other possibilities such as medication. This will depend on the individual's illness and their personal circumstances.

Medication

Certain antidepressant medications, known as selective serotonin reuptake inhibitors (SSRIs), have been shown to be beneficial to children and adolescents with severe depression.

It is very important that once started, medication should not be stopped suddenly. It may be needed for months or even years. Some people may, under medical supervision, be able to stop their medication when they have recovered and have felt well for a while.

Before starting the treatment or while on medication, a young person may need physical examinations and tests (e.g. blood tests). It is important that if the young person is prescribed medication, they are seen regularly by their doctor or psychiatrist.

There are side-effects to antidepressant medication, some of which can be quite serious. The psychiatrist will be able to advise you about what they are and what can be done to help. The risk of side-effects needs to be balanced against the risk of the damaging effects of the illness on a person's life.

No young person should be taking medication unless they are reviewed regularly by a health professional. This is to monitor the dose of the drug and to check for side-effects.

How else can I help?

Recognising and understanding your child's illness is a huge step in knowing how you can help. When your child becomes irritable or even does something risky, it is common for you to feel angry or upset. It is important that you try to remain calm and be honest about letting the child know what you feel and seek help.

Some children may be reluctant to talk to you about their problems, although they might talk to someone at school, a friend or their GP, or a professional for young people at a health centre or CAMHS. It is important to encourage them to talk to someone they can trust, as well as seeking professional help.

Having little chats, spending time with the young person watching TV, cooking and doing physical activities such as walking can help to lift their mood, even if they say they do not want to do it. A healthy diet and physical exercise can help improve their mood.

Useful websites

➲ **Young Minds**: www.youngminds.org.uk; free advice and support for parents worried about their children's behaviour, emotional problems and mental health. Parents' Helpline: 0808 802 5544.

➲ **Depression Alliance**: www.depressionalliance.org; help and information about depression, depression symptoms and self-help groups. Information line: 0845 123 23 20.

➲ **National Institute of Mental Health**: www.nimh.nih.gov; comprehensive information on mental health treatments and conditions across all ages.

Recommended reading

Other factsheets in this series: Psychosis, Bipolar disorder, CAMHS, Exercise and mental health

Rutter's Child and Adolescent Psychiatry (5th edn), edited by Sir Michael Rutter, Dorothy Bishop, Daniel Pine, et al. Wiley–Blackwell, 2008.

References

Bailey S, Shooter M (eds) *The Young Mind: An Essential Guide to Mental Health for Young Adults, Parents and Teachers*. RCPsych Publications, 2009.

Mufson L, Sills R. Interpersonal psychotherapy for depressed adolescents (IPT-A): an overview. *Nord J Psychiatry* 2006; 60: 431–7.

National Institute for Health and Clinical Health and Excellence. *Depression in Children and Young People* (CG28). NICE, 2005.

Notes

For a catalogue of public education materials or copies of our leaflets contact: Book Sales/Leaflets, The Royal College of Psychiatrists, 17 Belgrave Square, London SW1X 8PG. Email: leaflets@rcpsych.ac.uk, tel: 020 7235 2351 ext. 6146.

Revised by the Royal College of Psychiatrists' Child and Family Public Education Editorial Board. With grateful thanks to Dr Rasha Ravenscroft. This leaflet reflects the best possible evidence at the time of writing.

12 Worries and anxieties: helping children to cope
Information for parents, carers and anyone who works with young people

This is one in a series of factsheets for parents, teachers and anyone who works with young people, with practical, up-to-date information about mental health problems (emotional, behavioural and psychiatric disorders) that can affect children and young people.

This factsheet describes the different types of anxieties that children might feel and some of the reasons behind these. It also offers practical advice on how to deal with these worries and anxieties.

How common is anxiety in children?

Anxiety is one of the common mental health problems. Nearly 300 000 young people in Britain have an anxiety disorder. Lots of people, however, suffer in silence. It is important to recognise their problems and seek help, especially when it starts affecting their everyday life.

Growing up: different types of anxiety

Anxieties are grouped based on what the fear or worry is about. These groups are helpful in understanding what the difficulties are and how to treat them.

Why do children worry?

Children, like adults, have all sorts of strong feelings about what is happening to them. It's natural for them to feel fearful or worried from time to time. However, a small group of children and young people have severe anxiety which causes a lot of distress, and can seriously affect their everyday lives.

Fears and phobias

Young children often develop fears, for example of animals or of the dark. A phobia is an extreme fear which causes a lot of distress and affects the child's life significantly. For example, a fear of dogs is called a phobia if it means that a child refuses ever to go to the park to play.

Most children either grow out of their fears or learn to manage them with support and encouragement, but it is much more difficult to cope with a phobia without some extra help.

General anxiety

Some youngsters feel anxious most of the time for no apparent reason. It may be part of their temperament, or it may be part of a pattern of behaviour that is shared with other members of the family. If the anxiety becomes very severe, it can mean that the child will not want to go to school, cannot concentrate or learn, and is not confident with other people.

Separation anxiety

Worry about not being with a child's regular caregiver is a common experience for most children. It normally develops at 6 months, and can go on in some form during the pre-school years. It can make going to sleep, parents leaving for work, or settling at nursery or school very difficult at times. If it is extreme and affects the child's development, education and family life, it may be useful to get some additional help.

Social anxiety

It may be helpful to think of this as an extreme, sometimes disabling, type of shyness. It means that although children and young people are not affected in the company of family and people they know, they find it very worrying to be in other social situations. This means that they will usually avoid them. This causes problems for the child in making new friends or dealing with situations at school. Older children describe it as a fear of humiliation or embarrassment which leads them to avoiding social situations.

A small minority of children and young people may develop other specific types of anxiety, such as post-traumatic stress disorder (PTSD) or obsessive–compulsive disorder (OCD). Unlike young people and adults, it is extremely rare for children to have panic attacks.

What are the signs of anxiety?

Anxiety can cause both physical and emotional symptoms. This means it can affect how a person feels in their body and their health. Some of the symptoms are:

- feeling fearful or panicky
- feeling breathless, sweaty, or complaining of 'butterflies' or pains in the chest or stomach
- feeling tense, fidgety, using the toilet often.

These symptoms may come and go. Young children can't tell you that they are anxious. They become irritable, tearful and clingy, have difficulty sleeping, and can wake in the night or have bad dreams. Anxiety can even cause a child to develop a headache, a stomach ache or to feel sick.

What causes these worries and anxieties?

We do not really know what causes this condition. However, several things can contribute to anxiety in children, such as genes, where they live, having upsetting or traumatic experiences.

- Anxiety tends to run in families, so if someone in your family is known to worry a lot, their children may be more likely to worry as well. Some of this will be passed on in the genes, but children may also learn anxious behaviour from being around anxious people.
- Children who are bullied, lack friends or have trouble with their schoolwork often worry a lot.
- A child who has experienced a household fire or a burglary, a car accident or some other frightening or traumatic event, might suffer from anxiety afterwards. They might also develop PTSD.
- Children who have to cope with stressful situations such as bereavement, parental illness or divorce often become anxious and insecure. They may be able to manage one event, but may struggle to cope if several difficult things happen together, such as parents divorcing, moving home and changing school.
- Children need parents or caregivers to sooth them effectively. Young children can feel worried and anxious if they hear or see their parents arguing or fighting. If children sense their family or friends are anxious or harsh, it can make them feel more anxious. This leaves them feeling unsupported, insecure and lacking in confidence and can also be linked with separation anxiety.

Do children grow out of it?

Most children grow out of it, but a few continue being anxious and can sometimes become depressed as adults.

Even if they do not become anxious adults, anxiety can limit a young person's activities which can affect their development in the long term. Not going to school, for example, means missing out on education and making friends. Loneliness and lack of confidence can be long-term problems. The emotional effects of a traumatic experience can also be long-lasting.

David, 16, talks about his phobia of balloons as a younger child

'One of the worst things about my phobia was that I had to keep it secret. When my friends invited me to their birthdays, I had to say I was busy because I couldn't go anywhere near balloons.

I've always disliked balloons. I decided that my fear was out of control and I had to do something about it. I went with my mum to see our GP who sent me to a specialist. A couple of months later, we had the first of a course of eight cognitive–behavioural therapy sessions.

The therapist began by telling me that plenty of people have phobias and that balloon phobia even had a name ('globophobia'). It really helped to know that other people had the same problem. She asked me about my early life and tried to work out how my phobia had started. We talked about how I react to different stressful situations, marking how bad I'd feel on a scale of 1 to 10. She explained that my fast pulse rate, and my feeling hot and tense, and needing to escape were a normal response to stress. She taught me how to control my breathing, relax and talk to myself positively to control my anxiety.

Gradually, each week, I had harder things to do – at first just touching balloons, but by the end of the course – bursting them. On the way to the sessions I often got quite upset, because I knew I was going to have to face my greatest fear. It was hard work, and I nearly gave up.

I still don't like balloons, and would rather not have them near me, but thanks to the therapy, I can now deal with my fears.' ✪

What can I do to help?

A lot can be done to stop children being anxious. Parents and teachers can help by remembering that children, like adults, may get anxious about sudden change.

- It helps if you can prepare children in advance and explain what is going to happen and why.
- Regular routines around bedtime and getting ready for school can help very young children with separation anxiety.
- There may be books or games that can help children to understand upsetting things, such as serious illness, separation or bereavement.
- Children over the age of 5 often find it helpful to talk about their worries to an understanding adult, which could be someone outside the immediate family.
- Children may need comfort, reassurance and practical help with how to cope.

If your child is showing signs of anxiety, it is important that you can show them that you care and want to understand the reason why.

- Is there something going on in the family that could be causing worry?
- Are they picking up on your own worry?
- Is something happening at school or with friends?

All families have times when they have to deal with a lot of stress and worry. At times like these, you or your child might need extra help and support from friends, family members or others.

Where can I get help?

If your child is so anxious that they can't cope with ordinary day-to-day life, more specialist help is needed. Your GP will be able to advise you, and may suggest referral to the local child and adolescent mental health service (CAMHS). The type of specialist help offered here will depend on what is causing the anxiety. Basically, it will involve finding ways of overcoming the worries and building confidence step by step.

How is anxiety treated?

The type of specialist help offered will depend on what is causing the anxiety. Usually it will be a form of talking therapy such as cognitive–behavioural therapy (CBT) (see our factsheet on CBT). Cognitive–behavioural therapy can help the child understand what causes their anxiety and find strategies for coping. Parents are encouraged to be actively involved in helping their children manage their anxiety and are advised how to do this effectively.

Occasionally, a child might also be given a medicine to help if their anxiety problem has not got much better. A type of antidepressant, called an SSRI (selective serotonin reuptake inhibitor), is usually used.

Anxiety can be really difficult to live with for both the young person and family, but it is treatable.

Recommended reading

Other factsheets in this series: Obsessive–compulsive disorder, The emotional cost of bullying, Traumatic stress, Good parenting, CAMHS

National Institute for Health and Clinical Excellence: *Guide to Self-Help Resources for Generalised Anxiety Disorder* (2011). Available at http://guidance.nice.org.uk/CG113/SelfHelp.

Rays of Calm: Relaxation for Teenagers, by Christiane Kerr. This is a CD from the 'Calm for Kids' range created for teenagers. It talks through various relaxation techniques and visualisations designed to promote a sense of calm and well-being and to help teenagers deal with stress.

The Young Mind: An Essential Guide to Mental Health for Young Adults, Parents and Teachers, edited by Sue Bailey and Mike Shooter (2009) – an accessible, user-friendly handbook produced by the Royal College of Psychiatrists.

References

Baldwin DS, Anderson IM, Nutt DJ, et al. Evidence-based guidelines for the pharmacological treatment of anxiety disorders: recommendations from the British Association for Psychopharmacology. *J Psychopharmacol* 2005; 19: 567–96.

Green H, McGinnity A, Meltzer H, et al. *Mental Health of Children and Young People in Great Britain, 2004*. Office for National Statistics, 2005.

Ipser JC, Stein DJ, Hawkridge S, et al. Pharmacotherapy for anxiety disorders in children and adolescents. *Cochrane Database Syst Rev* 2009; 3: CD005170.

O'Kearney RT, Anstey KJ, von Sanden C, et al. Behavioural and cognitive behavioural therapy for obsessive compulsive disorder in children and adolescents. *Cochrane Database Syst Rev* 2006; 4: CD004856.

Useful websites

- **Anxiety UK**: www.anxietyuk.org.uk; charity providing information and support for people with anxiety problems.
- **TheSite.org**: www.thesite.org/healthandwellbeing; website by YouthNet UK, a charity that provides factsheets and articles on all the key issues facing young people.
- **Young Minds**: www.youngminds.org.uk; for any adult concerned about the emotions and behaviour of a child or young person. Parents' helpline: 0808 802 5544.
- **The Child Anxiety Network**: www.childanxiety.net; thorough, user-friendly information about child anxiety.
- **Website on social anxiety disorder**: www.social-anxiety.org
- **Youth Access**: http://youthaccess.org.uk; information, advice and counselling for young people in the UK. Has information on local services.

Notes

For a catalogue of public education materials or copies of our leaflets contact: Book Sales/Leaflets, The Royal College of Psychiatrists, 17 Belgrave Square, London SW1X 8PG. Email: leaflets@rcpsych.ac.uk, tel: 020 7235 2351 ext. 6146.

Revised by the Royal College of Psychiatrists' Child and Family Public Education Editorial Board. With grateful thanks to Dr Kashmeera Naidoo. This leaflet reflects the best possible evidence at the time of writing.

13 Divorce or separation of parents: the impact on children and adolescents
Information for parents, carers and anyone who works with young people

This is one in a series of factsheets for parents, teachers and anyone who works with young people, with practical, up-to-date information about mental health problems (emotional, behavioural and psychiatric disorders) that can affect children and young people.

This factsheet looks at the effect that divorce or separation of parents might have on children and young people, and offers practical advice on how to ease this.

How are children affected?

A child may feel:

- a sense of loss – separation from a parent can mean you lose not only your home, but your whole way of life
- different, with an unfamiliar family
- fearful about being left alone – if one parent can go, perhaps the other will do the same
- angry at one or both parents for the relationship breakdown
- worried about having caused the parental separation, guilty
- rejected and insecure
- torn between both parents.

These feelings are often made worse by the fact that many children have to move home and sometimes school when parents separate. Most families in this situation come under some financial strain, even if they did not have money worries before.

Even if the parental relationship had been very tense or violent, children may still have mixed feelings about the separation. Many children hold on to a wish that their parents may get back together.

Whatever has gone wrong in the relationship, both parents still have a very important part to play in their child's life.

What type of difficulties can children present with?

Emotional and behavioural problems in children are more common when their parents are fighting or separating. Children can become very insecure. Insecurity can cause them to behave like they are much younger: bed-wetting, being clingy, nightmares, worries or disobedience can all occur. This behaviour often happens before or after visits to the parent who is living apart from the family. Teenagers may show their distress by misbehaving or withdrawing into themselves. They may find it difficult to concentrate at school.

What can I do to help?

Parents who are separating can help their children. They should protect them from adult worries and responsibilities, and make it clear that the responsibility for what is happening is the parents' and not the child's.

How badly are children affected by divorce and separation in the UK?

Over half of couples divorcing in the UK in 2007 had at least one child aged under 16, which means that over 110 000 children were aged under 16 when their parents divorced; 20% of these children were under 5 years old. However, many more children go through parental separation each year and are not included in figures like this, as their parents were not married.

When parents no longer love each other and decide to live apart, a child can feel as if their world has been turned upside down. How upset a child feels can vary depending on how the parents separated, the age of the child, how much they understand, and the support they get from parents, family and friends.

Things that can help your child

- Be open and talk. Your child not only needs to know what is going on, but needs to feel that it's OK to ask questions.
- Reassure them that they will still have two parents who love them, and will continue to care for them.
- Make time to spend with your child.
- Be reliable about arrangements to see your child.
- Show that you are interested in your child's views, but make it clear that parents are responsible for the decisions.
- Carry on with the usual activities and routines such as seeing friends and members of the extended family.
- Make as few changes as possible. This will help your child feel that, in spite of the difficulties, loved ones still care about them and that life can be reasonably normal.

It is important not to pull your child into the conflict. The following tips may be useful.

Don't:

- ask your child to take sides: 'Who would you like to live with, darling?'
- ask your child what the other parent is doing
- use your child as a 'weapon' to get back at your ex-partner
- criticise your ex-partner in front of the child
- expect your child to take on the role of your ex-partner.

If you are finding it difficult to help your child cope, you may want to seek outside help. Your GP will be able to offer support and advice. Some families may need specialist help from the local child and adolescent mental health service (CAMHS). However, if managed sensitively, most children can adapt well to their new circumstances and do not have difficulties in the longer term.

Priya, 10, talks about her parents' divorce

'I can't remember when Mummy and Daddy ever really liked each other. Uma, my sister, said they did when she was little, before I was born, but that was a long time ago.

Daddy doesn't live with us anymore so we don't get to see him much. He's living with Nanny until he gets his own flat; but we can't stay over at Nanny's 'cos she says mean things about Mummy. Daddy rings us every night but sometimes Mummy will get cross with him and hang up before we've had a chance to talk.

I don't know why they don't like each other anymore. I sometimes think it's my fault as things seemed to go wrong after they had me. I think Uma blames me too. I can't speak to Mummy or Daddy about it 'cos I'm worried they'll say it is my fault. Even if they didn't, I probably wouldn't believe them.

I sometimes talk to Miss Hunter, my teacher, about my family. My friend Kate's parents split up a few years ago so she understands too. Her family all went for some sort of counselling together which Kate said was really good as it made them all listen to each other and talk without shouting. Kate hoped the counselling would mean her Daddy would move back home, but it didn't work out that way.

I think my family should have counselling too, not to get Mummy and Daddy back together (I don't think that'll ever happen), but it might make them listen to me and Uma a bit more. Especially now they are talking about where we are going to live and how often we see Daddy.

Mummy said we might have to move house which might mean changing schools. Them splitting up doesn't just mean Daddy doesn't live with us anymore; our whole lives are different. I don't think they get how hard this is for us.' ✪

Useful websites

- ➲ **The Children's Society**: www.childrenssociety.org.uk; produces a series of leaflets for children and parents.

- ➲ **Citizens Advice Bureau**: www.citizensadvice.org.uk; your local branch is listed in the telephone directory.

- ➲ **Divorce Aid**: www.divorceaid.co.uk; run by an independent group of professionals, the website provides advice, support and information on all aspects of divorce. It has specialised sections for both young children and teenagers, enabling them to recognise and deal with emotions that arise from separation and divorce.

- ➲ **Money Advice Service**: www.moneyadviceservice.org.uk; information and advice on the financial aspects of divorce, separation or civil partnership dissolution, including an interactive calculator to help manage finances, work out what you have and owe, and consider how you might split what you have.

- ➲ **National Family Mediation**: www.nfm.org.uk; an organisation specifically set up to help families who are separating. It has a useful booklist, which includes books for children of different ages.

- ➲ **Family Lives**: http://familylives.org.uk/; offers help and advice to parents on bringing up children and teenagers. Helpline: 0808 800 2222.

- ➲ **Relate**: www.relate.org.uk; helps couples with relationship difficulties.

- ➲ **Action for Children**: www.itsnotyourfault.org; supports families through divorce, bereavement and children's behavioural problems.

Recommended reading

Other factsheets in this series: Worries and anxieties, CAMHS

Rutter's Child and Adolescent Psychiatry (5th edn), edited by Sir Michael Rutter, Dorothy Bishop, Daniel Pine, et al. Wiley–Blackwell, 2008.

The Young Mind: An Essential Guide to Mental Health for Young Adults, Parents and Teachers, edited by Sue Bailey and Mike Shooter (2009) – an accessible, user-friendly handbook produced by the Royal College of Psychiatrists.

References

Lee CM, Bax KA. Children's reactions to parental separation and divorce. *Paediatrics Child Health* 2000; 5: 217–8.

Rutter M, Bishop D, Pine D, et al (eds) *Rutter's Child and Adolescent Psychiatry* (5th edn). Wiley–Blackwell, 2008.

Notes

For a catalogue of public education materials or copies of our leaflets contact: Book Sales/Leaflets, The Royal College of Psychiatrists, 17 Belgrave Square, London SW1X 8PG. Email: leaflets@rcpsych.ac.uk, tel: 020 7235 2351 ext. 6146.

Revised by the Royal College of Psychiatrists' Child and Family Public Education Editorial Board. With grateful thanks to Dr Margaret Bamforth. This leaflet reflects the best possible evidence at the time of writing.

14 Death in the family: helping children to cope

Information for parents, carers and anyone who works with young people

This is one in a series of factsheets for parents, teachers and anyone who works with young people, with practical, up-to-date information about mental health problems (emotional, behavioural and psychiatric disorders) that can affect children and young people.

This factsheet looks at how a death in the family may affect a child or young person, and offers advice on how to cope with this situation.

How does a child respond to death?

How children react to death depends on a number of factors.

- How close the person who died was to the child, and the family, is important and how involved that person was in their lives.
- Whether the death was sudden or expected (a relief from suffering or a crushing blow). How traumatic it was can have an impact on how children cope with it.
- The circumstances of the death also affect the impact it has on the child. Each family responds in its own way to death. Religion and culture will have an important influence on what happens.

Other factors that can make a big difference from the child's point of view are:

- the effect of grief on other family members, especially if they are not able to cope with giving the child the care they need
- how much practical support is available to help the family cope.

> ### Children and bereavement
>
> Everyone can experience grief when they lose someone close to them. They may need to spend a period of time in bereavement coming to terms with the grief.
>
> Death in the family affects everyone. Children in particular need to be thought about even if it is a difficult time for the whole family.

How do children of different ages understand death?

The child's age and level of understanding can affect how the death affects their life.

Infants may feel the loss because it affects the way in which they are looked after and their daily routine. They are very sensitive to the unhappy feelings of those around them, and may become anxious, difficult to settle and more needy of attention.

Pre-school children usually see death as temporary and reversible, a belief reinforced by cartoon characters that 'die' and 'come to life' again.

Children from about the age of 5 are able to understand basic facts about death:

- it happens to all living things
- it has a cause
- it involves permanent separation.

They can also understand that dead people do not need to eat or drink and do not see, hear, speak or feel.

Most children get angry and worried, as well as sad, about death. Anger is a natural reaction to the loss of someone who was essential to the child's sense of stability and safety. A child may show this anger in boisterous play, by being irritable, or in nightmares. Anxiety is shown in 'babyish' talk and behaviours that can include demanding food, comfort and cuddles.

Young children believe that they cause what happens around them. They may worry that they caused the death by being naughty.

Teenagers are able to understand death much more like adults and are very aware of the feelings of others. They may find it difficult to put their feelings into words, and may not show their feelings openly, for fear of upsetting others.

How do I help a child to cope with death?

Being aware of how children normally respond to death makes it easier for an adult to help. It also makes it easier to notice if a child is struggling.

Help in early stages after death

Adults sometimes try to protect children from pain by not telling them what has happened. Experience shows that children benefit from knowing the **truth** at an early stage. They may even want to see the dead relative. The closer the relationship, the more important this is.

Adults can also help children to cope by **listening** to the child's experience of the death, answering their questions and reassuring them. Children often worry that they will be abandoned by loved ones, or fear that they are to blame for the death. If they can talk about this, and express themselves through play, they can cope better and are less likely to have emotional disturbances later in life.

Young children often find it difficult to recall **memories** of a dead person without first being reminded of them. They can be very upset by not having these memories. A photograph can be a great source of comfort.

Children usually find it helpful to be included in family activities, such as attending the **funeral**. Thought should be given as to how to support and prepare a child for this. A child who is frightened about attending a funeral should not be forced to go. However, except for very young children, it is usually important to find a way to enable them to say goodbye. For example, they can light a candle, say a prayer or visit the grave.

Helping later on

Once children accept the death, they are likely to display their feelings of sadness, anger and anxiety on and off, sometimes over a long period of time, and often at unexpected moments. The surviving relatives should spend as much time as possible with the child, making it clear that they can show their feelings openly, without fear of upsetting others.

Sometimes a child may 'forget' that the family member has died, or persist in the belief that they are still alive. This is normal in the first few weeks following a death, but may cause problems if it continues.

What are signs that a child is not coping?

Some of the warning signs that your child may need more help include:

- a long period of sadness or depression, with a reduced interest in daily activities
- withdrawing from friends
- inability to sleep, loss of appetite, prolonged fear of being alone
- a sharp drop in school performance, or refusal to attend school
- acting like a much younger child for a long time
- denying that the family member has died
- imitating the dead person all the time
- talking repeatedly about wanting to join the dead person.

These warning signs mean that professional help may be needed. Your GP will be able to offer you help and advice, and can refer you and your child to specialists who can provide bereavement counselling or to your local child and adolescent mental health service (CAMHS). They can help the child to accept the death, and also assist the family to find ways of helping the child through the mourning process.

Josh, 17, talks about the loss of his father

'Mum and Dad separated when I was a 3-month-old baby, but I always spent every other weekend with Dad. I loved staying with him even though the flat was always messy and he spent most of the weekend down the pub. But I had my mates upstairs, two brothers, who became my best friends.

One weekend Dad complained of terrible pains in his chest and my friend's mother called the ambulance – Dad nearly died in hospital and I was with him. I wasn't allowed to tell Mum about it because Dad was worried that I wouldn't be able to see him again. When Mum picked me up from hospital, Dad told her that he had had an ulcer which had burst.

Dad died not long after that, funnily enough on Father's Day. He died of alcoholism – I was 8. I find it difficult to talk about him, even to this day, because Mum and Dad were divorced and she was still angry with him. I also felt very guilty that I wasn't with him as I am sure that I could have saved him. I get very down about that.

When my school friends found out that he had died, they didn't know what to say to me and somehow I always felt different to the others. Even if their parents were separated or divorced, they still had two parents and I only had one.

I have two framed pictures of my dad in my bedroom, but I have forgotten his face and this makes me feel very guilty. Sometimes I dream of him, but he will always be the 46-year-old man that I loved and knew – he will never grow old.

Recently, Dad's brother died and I met up with all the grandparents, aunts, uncles, nieces and nephews from his side of the family. It was wonderful to speak about him openly and remember him.' ✪

Recommended reading

Other factsheets in this series:
Worries and anxieties, CAMHS

The Young Mind: An Essential Guide to Mental Health for Young Adults, Parents and Teachers, edited by Sue Bailey and Mike Shooter (2009) – an accessible, user-friendly handbook produced by the Royal College of Psychiatrists.

When Someone Very Special Dies – Children can Learn to Cope with Grief, by M. Heegard. Woodland Press, 1991.

References

Melvin D, Lukeman D. Bereavement: a framework for those working with children. *Clin Child Psychol Psychiatry* 2000; 5: 521–39.

Rutter M, Bishop D, Pine D, et al (eds) *Rutter's Child and Adolescent Psychiatry* (5th edn). Wiley–Blackwell, 2008.

Schultz K. Bereaved children. *Can Fam Physician* 1999; 45: 2914–21.

Useful websites

➲ **Cruse Bereavement Care**: www.crusebereavementcare. org.uk; promotes the well-being of bereaved people and helps understand their grief and cope with their loss. It also has a website, helpline and email specifically for young people experiencing bereavement: www.rd4u.org.uk, email: info@rd4u. org.uk, helpline: 0808 808 1677.

➲ **Winston's Wish**: www.winstonswish.org.uk; supports bereaved children, young people and families. Helpline: 08452 03 04 05.

➲ **Child Bereavement Charity**: www.childbereavement.org.uk; a national charity which works to help bereaved families where a baby or child has died, or where children are bereaved of someone important in their lives.

Notes

....

....

....

....

....

....

....

....

....

....

....

For a catalogue of public education materials or copies of our leaflets contact: Book Sales/Leaflets, The Royal College of Psychiatrists, 17 Belgrave Square, London SW1X 8PG. Email: leaflets@rcpsych.ac.uk, tel: 020 7235 2351 ext. 6146.

Revised by the Royal College of Psychiatrists' Child and Family Public Education Editorial Board. With grateful thanks to Dr Fareeha Amber Sadiq. This leaflet reflects the best possible evidence at the time of writing.

This is one in a series of factsheets for parents, teachers and anyone who works with young people, with practical, up-to-date information about mental health problems (emotional, behavioural and psychiatric disorders) that can affect children and young people.

This factsheet looks in detail at what bullying is and how it can affect young people. It also gives advice for parents and teachers about how they can help a young person who is being bullied.

What does it mean that someone is being bullied?

Children who bully may:

- hit or punch another child
- kick them or trip them up
- take or spoil their things
- call them names
- tease them
- give them nasty looks
- threaten them
- make racist remarks about them
- spread nasty rumours or stories about them
- not let them join in play or games
- not talk to them – 'send him to Coventry'
- sending repeated false or obscene messages on the phone or internet/social networking sites.

What is bullying?

Bullying happens when a child is picked on by another child or group of children. It is hurtful and deliberate. Victims find it difficult to defend themselves. Bullying usually happens again and again, and can go on for a long time unless something is done about it.

It can happen in many different ways which include physical, verbal or emotional bullying.

How common is bullying?

Bullying is very common and can happen in all schools. Surveys in England have shown that half of primary school pupils and one in ten secondary school pupils are being bullied.

Why does it happen?

There is no single reason why some children become bullies or victims. Children who are aggressive are more likely to become bullies. They pick on children who appear different in some way – those who are quiet, shy, alone at playtime, and unable to defend themselves. Children who have an illness or disability or who are obese are also more likely to be bullied.

What effects does bullying have?

Being bullied can seriously affect a child's physical and mental health. This can include:

- feeling sad and lonely
- lacking confidence and feeling bad about themselves
- becoming depressed
- complaining of various physical symptoms, such as headaches or stomach aches
- worrying and trying to avoid going to school.

These problems can carry on long after the bullying has stopped.

Who and what can help?

Parents

- **Be open to the possibility that your child might be being bullied.** Some parents may not think of bullying as a possible reason for their child's distress.

- **Listen.** One of the most important things you can do is to listen to your child if they say they are being bullied. It can be very difficult for them to talk to anyone about it.

- **Take your child seriously.** Many children suffer in silence for a long time before they tell anyone. They may be ashamed, embarrassed, and may believe that they deserve it. Many children are frightened of telling someone what is happening because they fear the bullies will find out and hurt them even more. It can take great courage to tell an adult.

- **Do not blame the child.** Being bullied is not their fault (although they may think it is).

- **Reassure** them that they were right to tell you.

- **Do not promise to keep the bullying a secret.** Something must be done about it. Reassure your child that you, and the teachers, will make sure that things do not get worse because they have told you. Tell the school so they can stop it. Teachers don't always know that a child is being bullied. Find out whether there is an anti-bullying programme in the school.

- **Talk with your child and work out ways of solving the problem.** Include your child in decisions about how to tackle the problem. For example, work out some practical ways for them to stop the bullying. You might discuss what they should say back if they are called names, or where it's safe to go at playtime.

School

Bullying can happen in any school, so it is important that each school has an effective anti-bullying programme. They should make it clear that they won't allow bullying or aggressive behaviour. Schools that have these policies and who take every incident of bullying seriously, tend to have less bullying.

Every school can obtain an anti-bullying pack from the Department for Education. There are a number of agencies that can offer advice and help in how to set up effective programmes (see 'Useful websites' and 'Recommended reading' at the end of this factsheet).

Other professionals who can help

Children whose health has been affected by bullying may benefit from some specialist help from their GP, school nurse, a social worker or an educational psychologist who will be able to offer help and advice. Children with emotional problems quite often need these to be treated directly, even if the school has managed to stop the bullying. Your GP can refer your child to a child and adolescent mental health service (CAMHS).

Jax, 14

'I don't know whether it has ever happened to you? It started when Justine came into our class. I was friends with Jo and Justine wanted to hang round with us. It was OK at first, but then she and Jo began laughing about things and I didn't know what was funny. They had secrets they wouldn't tell me. They started nicking my things and pretending I had lost them. I stopped hanging around with them and sat next to Lucy in English and Science. She was my friend from primary school.

Then they started spreading rumours about me. They said I was a slag and slept with Pete. They said I was pregnant. They started sending me horrible text messages. They got everyone against me. I didn't want to tell my mum but she found out when I told her because she found me crying in my room.

I wouldn't go to school. Mum went to school and spoke to Miss Ratcliffe but she said they, the teachers, hadn't seen anything and they couldn't do anything about it. I got really down. My mum went to school and got angry because I was missing so much school. They got everyone together and changed my form. They also gave me a mentor. Things are better now but I still don't speak to Jo and Justine – although they aren't friends anymore.' ✪

Recommended reading

Other factsheets in this series:
Coping with stress, Depression,
When bad things happen, CAMHS

Preventing and Tackling Bullying – Advice for School Leaders, Staff and Governing Bodies, a booklet produced by the Department for Education, 2011.

The Young Mind: An Essential Guide to Mental Health for Young Adults, Parents and Teachers, edited by Sue Bailey and Mike Shooter (2009) – an accessible, user-friendly handbook produced by the Royal College of Psychiatrists.

References

Bond L, Carlin JB, Thomas L, et al. Does bullying cause emotional problems? A prospective study of young teenagers. *BMJ* 2001; 323: 480–4.

Gini G, Pozzoli T. Association between bullying and psychosomatic problems: a meta-analysis. *Pediatrics* 2009; 123: 1059–65.

National Institute for Health and Clinical Excellence. *Promoting Children's Social and Emotional Wellbeing in Primary Education* (PH12). NICE, 2008.

National Institute for Health and Clinical Excellence. *Promoting Young People's Social and Emotional Wellbeing in Secondary Education* (PH20). NICE, 2009.

Vreeman RC, Carroll AE. A systematic review of school-based interventions to prevent bullying. *Arch Pediatrics Adolesc Med* 2007; 161: 78–88.

Useful websites

- **ChildLine**: www.childline.org.uk; provides a free and confidential telephone service for children: 0800 1111.

- **Kidscape**: www.kidscape.org.uk; provides advice, runs training courses and produces helpful booklets and information about bullying.

- **Bullying UK**: www.bullying.co.uk; part of Family Lives, a national charity providing help and support in all aspects of family life. Helpline: 0808 800 2222.

- **Beatbullying**: www.beatbullying.org; a bullying prevention charity working directly with children and young people.

- **The Anti-Bullying Alliance (ABA)**: www.anti-bullyingalliance. org.uk; brings together over 130 organisations into one network to develop and share good practice across the whole range of bullying issues.

Notes

....
....
....
....
....
....
....
....
....
....
....

16 Traumatic stress in children
Information for parents, carers and anyone who works with young people

This is one in a series of factsheets for parents, teachers and anyone who works with young people, with practical, up-to-date information about mental health problems (emotional, behavioural and psychiatric disorders) that can affect children and young people.

This factsheet describes the causes and symptoms of traumatic stress and provides practical advice on how to get help.

What are the signs of traumatic stress?

Individual children react in different ways to traumatic events. How they react may also depend on their age.

Immediately after the traumatic event, children may find it hard to sleep and have bad dreams and nightmares. Sometimes, the effects may not appear for days or weeks. Children may, however:

- become fearful, clingy and anxious about being separated from their parents
- start bed-wetting and thumb-sucking again
- become preoccupied with thoughts and memories of the event
- be unable to concentrate
- be irritable and disobedient
- complain of physical symptoms such as headaches and stomach aches.

All these are normal reactions to an extremely frightening event. With help and support from the people close to them, children begin to get over the shock in a few days, and usually recover after a few weeks.

What is traumatic stress?

Children, like adults, sometimes experience or witness something extremely frightening and dangerous, such as a road accident, a serious injury or a crime. This can cause a traumatic stress reaction which affects the way the child thinks, feels and behaves. Children can be as severely affected as adults. If you recognise it, you will be better able to help your child to recover, and also know when to seek professional help.

What are the long-term effects of traumatic stress?

Sometimes a child has feelings of depression and anxiety that go on for several weeks and may get worse. If they continue for a long period of time, it is likely that the child may need some help to feel better.

If the traumatic experience was so bad that the child was in danger of being killed or seriously injured, they may have felt terrified, horrified and helpless. Post-traumatic stress disorder (PTSD) might follow a dreadful experience of this sort. It is difficult, however, to make a diagnosis in a child under the age of 7 years.

Some of the typical signs of PTSD

- 'Flashbacks' of the event. For a few moments, it seems as though you are reliving the experience in your mind, like watching an action-replay. This can be distressing and frightening, particularly for children.
- Deliberately avoiding thoughts or feelings about the traumatic experience. If the child has been in a car crash, they may avoid roads or even TV programmes about cars because it reminds them of the accident.
- Sleeping badly.
- Being easily startled and appearing frightened at the slightest noise.

These reactions can go on for months and can interfere considerably with a child's daily living. They may be unable to enjoy playing or find it difficult to concentrate on their schoolwork. Occasionally, these problems can continue as the child grows into adulthood.

What can help?

The best approach, immediately after a traumatic event, is to **accept** that a child will be distressed – this is normal. At this stage, parents can help greatly by letting their child talk about the event if they want to, or helping them to relive it in games and drawings.

Leaving children alone 'to forget things' does not help. **Talking** can help children to adjust. It helps them to make sense of what has happened, to feel less alone with their worries and to regain a sense of control. However, forcing someone to talk about it when they don't want to does not seem to be helpful.

If you have been involved in the traumatic event, you may also be distressed. It is usually better to **admit** to your children that you are feeling sad and upset. At the same time, you need to make it clear that you don't expect them to look after your feelings. If you recognise that you have symptoms of PTSD then get help. Your child will manage their feelings and emotions better if you are not feeling fearful or anxious yourself.

Sometimes, children find it easier to talk to other adults rather than their parents. **Professional help** may be needed to help them get back to normal more quickly, and to prevent or reduce the harmful effects of prolonged stress reactions.

When should I seek help?

Ask for help if:

- the child's upset feelings and behaviour seem to be getting worse
- the signs of extreme stress last for longer than about a month
- worries prevent you, your child or your family getting on with normal, everyday life
- the child has symptoms of PTSD that go on for longer than a month.

Where can I get help?

If you are concerned about your child at any time following a traumatic event, consult your GP, who will be able to offer you help and support. If problems continue, the doctor may suggest extra help from the local child and adolescent mental health service (CAMHS).

If you have been involved directly in a community disaster, special support services may be arranged. Do not hesitate to make contact with them if you want to talk over your worries.

Kylie, 11

'We had a car crash 3 months ago. This other car was on the wrong side of the road and ran into us. Luckily, we were OK, but the man in the other car was hurt really badly.

At first, I was still myself afterwards. But after a few weeks, I stopped sleeping properly. I'd have really bad dreams about the crash; I'd see the other car all mashed up and the man inside covered in blood. Sometimes, I'd see the same thing but while I was awake. I couldn't sleep on my own anymore and had to go into Mum and Dad's bed 'cos I was so scared; I hadn't done that since I was tiny.

I became really frightened, especially about cars and roads. I couldn't go anywhere in the car, even if it was Mum or Dad driving, and then even walking on the pavement felt scary. It meant it was really difficult to get to school and I missed a lot of my lessons.

Mum spoke to my head of year, and took me to see the doctor. The doctor said she thought I'd become really frightened because of the crash and that talking to someone might help. She sent me to see Clare; Mum says she's a psychologist. I've seen Clare six times now, I go every week. Sometimes Mum and Dad come too. We talk and also do stuff outside, practical stuff Clare says will help me be less frightened about cars and roads. I do get scared when we go out of her office and on to the pavement, but she talks me through it and we stay outside until I feel OK again.

I've not been in a car yet – that feels too scary at the moment, but I am doing better than I was, so it might not be too long. My teachers have given me work to do at home and I'm planning to try to go back to school after half term, maybe just a few hours each day at first. Clare says it's better to do things like that step by step.' ✪

Recommended reading

Other factsheets in this series: Death in the family, Divorce or separation of parents, Domestic violence, Child abuse and neglect, CAMHS

The Young Mind: An Essential Guide to Mental Health for Young Adults, Parents and Teachers, edited by Sue Bailey and Mike Shooter (2009) – an accessible, user-friendly handbook produced by the Royal College of Psychiatrists.

References

Rutter M, Bishop D, Pine D, et al (eds) *Rutter's Child and Adolescent Psychiatry* (5th edn). Wiley–Blackwell, 2008.

Useful websites

➲ **Cruse Bereavement Care**: www.crusebereavementcare. org.uk; promotes the well-being of bereaved people and helps understand their grief and cope with their loss. It also has a website, helpline and email specifically for young people experiencing bereavement: www.rd4u.org.uk, email: info@rd4u. org.uk, helpline: 0808 808 1677.

➲ **The Samaritans**: www.samaritans.org.uk; 24-hour service offering confidential emotional support to anyone who is in crisis. Helpline: 08457 909090 (UK), 1850 609090 (Northern Ireland), email: jo@samaritans.org

➲ **Victim Support**: www.victimsupport.org; gives free and confidential help to victims of crime, witnesses, their family, friends and anyone else affected across England and Wales. Helpline: 0845 30 30 900.

Notes

....
....
....
....
....
....
....
....
....

For a catalogue of public education materials or copies of our leaflets contact: Book Sales/Leaflets, The Royal College of Psychiatrists, 17 Belgrave Square, London SW1X 8PG. Email: leaflets@rcpsych.ac.uk, tel: 020 7235 2351 ext. 6146.

Revised by the Royal College of Psychiatrists' Child and Family Public Education Editorial Board. With grateful thanks to Dr Margaret Bamforth. This leaflet reflects the best possible evidence at the time of writing.

17 Domestic violence: its effects on children
Information for parents, carers and anyone who works with young people

This is one in a series of factsheets for parents, teachers and anyone who works with young people, with practical, up-to-date information about mental health problems (emotional, behavioural and psychiatric disorders) that can affect children and young people.

This factsheet looks at the effects that domestic violence can have on children and offers advice about how to help them.

Who are the abusers and victims?

Although a man abusing a woman is recognised more often, the adults may be of either gender or any sexuality. It can happen among people of any class, religion, race, occupation or age.

It is common thinking that alcohol and mental illness can cause a person to be violent. Alcohol does not cause domestic violence, but there is evidence that where domestic violence exists, alcohol is often present. Most people who are mentally ill are not violent.

Anyone can be a victim of domestic violence. Children, even pets, can be affected. People with mental illness are more likely to be the victims of violence than perpetrators of violence.

How are children involved?

In relationships where there is domestic violence, children witness about three-quarters of the abusive incidents. About half the children in these families have themselves been badly hit or beaten. Sexual and emotional abuse is also more likely to happen in these families.

How are children affected?

It is very upsetting for children to see one of their parents (or carers) abusing or attacking the other. They often show signs of great distress.

- Younger children may become **anxious**. They can complain of tummy aches or start to wet their bed. They may find it difficult to sleep, have temper tantrums and start to behave as if they are much younger than they are.

- Older children react differently. Boys seem to express their distress much more outwardly. They may become **aggressive** and **disobedient**. Sometimes, they start to use violence like **bullying** to try and solve problems, and may copy the behaviour they see within the family. Older boys may play truant and start to use alcohol or **drugs**.

- Girls are more likely to keep their distress inside. They may become **withdrawn** from other people, and become anxious or **depressed**. They may think badly of themselves and complain of vague physical symptoms. They are more likely to have an **eating disorder** or to **harm themselves** by taking overdoses or cutting themselves.

- Children with these problems often do badly at school. They may refuse to go to school. They may also get symptoms of **post-traumatic stress disorder**, for example, have nightmares and flashbacks, and be easily startled.

What is domestic violence?

The term domestic violence or domestic abuse is used to describe any incident of threatening behaviour, violence or abuse between adults, who are/have been family members or living at the family home. These incidents may be psychological, physical (including throwing objects), sexual, emotional (including verbal threats, controlling behaviour) or financial.

Abuse can also happen on mobile phones, on the internet and on social networking sites.

> **Matty, 13, talks about the problems with her family**
>
> 'It's only in the past year or so that I began to think that a family could be a good place to be… a home. I'm the eldest child in the family and I took a lot of my dad's anger. I know my mum wasn't always a saint – she could really wind him up – in fact she does it to me sometimes and then I get terrified that I'll react like him.
>
> Anyway, sometimes they would just argue and shout, but then I saw what he could do when he lost it. I had to take mum to hospital once and it was just horrible. In fact, I remember being amazed how she looked almost normal when they'd cleaned her up. But seeing it, or even worse, just hearing it was… don't know… I couldn't bear it, and I wanted to kill him. I couldn't, I know – even if I was strong enough – so I just used to hold on to the little ones and sort of hide with them till it was over.
>
> But it did get so difficult. I didn't want to go home after school, so I'd stay out late, sometimes with my mates. Then my mum started saying I was just like him. That was the worst time ever.
>
> One day my mum spoke to someone on a helpline. After that, they had a big row and then he left home. Things sort of calmed down, but I was still scared that he would come back or I'd be like him. Then we had this counsellor who talked to my mum, and me and my sisters together. Somehow it all began to seem better and I felt it was possible to move on.' ✪

Are there any long-term effects?

Children who have witnessed violence are more likely to become abusive or a victim themselves. Children tend to copy the behaviour of their parents. Boys can learn from their fathers to be violent to women. Girls can learn from their mothers that violence is to be expected, and something you just have to put up with.

Some children appear 'resilient', are able to withstand and are less affected by the domestic violence. Children don't always repeat the same pattern when they grow up. Many children don't like what they see, and try very hard not to make the same mistakes as their parents. Even so, children from violent families often grow up feeling anxious and depressed, and find it difficult to get on with other people.

What can help?

- **Talking about it**

  Open communication about the problem is helpful, much more than trying to hide it. Children are able to cope better and recover when they get the right help and support, for example from other family members, peers or school. Some children would find it helpful to speak to a professional (e.g. a trained counsellor).

- **Confiding in someone**

  It is not uncommon for victims of domestic violence to take a long time to recognise what is happening. Even when they do, it can feel extremely difficult to take any action about it. Speaking to someone they can trust or to a professional can help them in this process.

- **Getting professional help**

  Professionals such as doctors, nurses, teachers and social workers should be able to talk to you and your child and offer the help and advice needed. In some areas, local domestic violence support may be available.

- **Staying safe**

  Remember, it is important to keep yourself and your children safe. Asking for help early and when in crisis is important. Domestic violence is a crime – when required, you should call the police.

- **Practical issues**

  In the long term, practical help may be needed from professionals such as social workers or solicitors. They will be able to help with finding a place to live, dealing with money problems, and making contact and school arrangements for the children.

Useful websites

- **NSPCC**: www.nspcc.org.uk; the NSPCC Helpline provides advice and support to adults who are concerned about the safety or welfare of a child. Helpline: 0808 800 5000.
- **ChildLine**: www.childline.org.uk; free, confidential helpline dedicated to children and young people: 0800 1111.
- **Women's Aid**: www.womensaid.org.uk; national charity working to end domestic violence against women and children. Helpline: 0808 2000 247.
- **The Hideout**: www.thehideout.org.uk; Women's Aid have created this space to help children and young people to understand domestic abuse and how to take positive action.
- **The Samaritans**: www.samaritans.org.uk; a 24-hour service offering confidential emotional support to anyone who is in crisis. Helpline: 08457 909090 (UK), 1850 609090 (Northern Ireland), email: jo@samaritans.org
- **Victim Support**: www.victimsupport.org; free and confidential help to victims of crime, witnesses, their family, friends and anyone else affected across England and Wales. Support line: 0845 30 30 900.
- **Respect**: www.respect.uk.net; UK membership association lobbying for domestic violence perpetrator programmes and associated support services. Helpline for perpetrators: 0808 802 4040.

Recommended reading

Other factsheets in this series: Traumatic stress in children, Child abuse and neglect, CAMHS

References

Department of Health. *Improving Safety, Reducing Harm: Children, Young People and Domestic Violence. A Practical Toolkit for Frontline Practitioners*. Department of Health, 2009.

EACH. *Asian Women, Domestic Violence and Mental Health: A Toolkit for Health Professionals*. Government Office for London, 2009.

Galvani S. *Grasping the Nettle: Alcohol and Domestic Violence* (revised). Alcohol Concern, 2010.

Rutter M, Bishop D, Pine D, et al (eds) *Rutter's Child and Adolescent Psychiatry* (5th edn). Wiley–Blackwell, 2008.

Scottish Government. *A Review of Literature on Effective Interventions that Prevent and Respond to Harm Against Adults*. Scottish Executive, 2007.

Notes

For a catalogue of public education materials or copies of our leaflets contact: Book Sales/Leaflets, The Royal College of Psychiatrists, 17 Belgrave Square, London SW1X 8PG. Email: leaflets@rcpsych.ac.uk, tel: 020 7235 2351 ext. 6146.

Revised by the Royal College of Psychiatrists' Child and Family Public Education Editorial Board. With grateful thanks to Dr Vasu Balaguru. This leaflet reflects the best possible evidence at the time of writing.

18 Child abuse and neglect: the emotional effect
Information for parents, carers and anyone who works with young people

This is one in a series of factsheets for parents, teachers and anyone who works with young people, with practical, up-to-date information about mental health problems (emotional, behavioural and psychiatric disorders) that can affect children and young people.

This factsheet looks at what child abuse is and the harm it can cause, and offers practical help about how to detect it and where to get help.

Who abuses children?

Children are usually abused by someone in their immediate family circle. This can include parents, brothers or sisters, babysitters or other familiar adults. It is quite unusual for strangers to be involved.

How can you tell if a child is being abused?

Children may present with a variety of difficulties and behaviours depending on where, when and what type of abuse they have experienced.

It can be hard to detect long-standing abuse by an adult the child is close to. It is often very difficult for the child to tell anyone about it, as the abuser may have threatened to hurt them if they tell anybody. A child may not say anything because they think it is their fault, that no one will believe them or that they will be teased or punished. The child may even love the abusing adult. They want the abuse to stop, but they don't want the adult to go to prison or for the family to break up.

Some of the signs of abuse are described below.

Physically abused children may:

- be watchful, cautious or wary of adults
- be unable to play and be spontaneous
- be aggressive or abusive
- bully other children or be bullied themselves
- be unable to concentrate, underachieve at school and avoid activities that involve removal of clothes, e.g. sports
- have temper tantrums and behave thoughtlessly
- lie, steal, play truant from school and get into trouble with the police
- find it difficult to trust other people and make friends.

Sexually abused children may:

- suddenly behave differently when the abuse starts
- think badly of themselves
- not look after themselves
- use sexual talk or ideas in their play that you would usually see only in someone much older
- withdraw into themselves or be secretive
- underachieve at school
- start wetting or soiling themselves
- be unable to sleep
- behave in an inappropriately seductive or flirtatious way

What is child abuse?

All parents upset their children sometimes. Saying 'no' and managing difficult behaviour is an essential part of parenting. Tired or stressed parents can lose control and can do or say something they regret, and may even hurt the child. If it is severe or happens often, it can seriously harm the child. That is why abuse is defined in law. The Children Act 1989 states that abuse should be considered to have happened when someone's actions have caused a child to suffer 'significant harm' to their health or development.

'Significant harm' means that someone is:

- punishing a child too much
- hitting or shaking a child
- constantly criticising, threatening or rejecting a child
- sexually interfering with or assaulting a child
- not looking after a child – not giving them enough to eat, ignoring them, not playing or talking with them or not making sure that they are safe.

Kate, 16, talks about her abuse

'It started when I was about 8 and me and my sister went to stay with my aunt and uncle. My sister, aunt and cousins went out, but I didn't feel well so I stayed behind. My uncle said he had a game that would make me feel better. He said it was a special game that we could play with my cousin's Barbie doll. In the game, Barbie got married and then went on her honeymoon – he said on a honeymoon people do special things and he could show me what they were, but I mustn't tell anyone because I'd get into serious trouble.

He took Barbie's clothes off and I don't really remember what he did next. He said he could show me how to play this game – that it would make him happy. It's really hard to talk about what happened next. Then he made me promise I wouldn't tell anyone, he said people wouldn't understand and would get angry with me. Then he gave me some sweets. After that, whenever I went to visit something would happen.

In the beginning he was quite nice to me and although I didn't want it to happen, I didn't want to upset him. I'd pretend it wasn't happening.

Then I began to get scared of him, he'd get angry. It got harder to pretend it wasn't happening and I thought about it a lot, I felt really sad. My mum asked if anything was wrong but I couldn't tell her – he said she would be angry with me and that anyway no one would believe me. I felt so upset and scared and trapped – I couldn't tell anyone and couldn't stop it.

I started to cut myself. I told my friend at school, she said she'd seen a programme when a girl rang ChildLine. She helped me find the number and let me use her mum's phone.

They talked to me and that made me feel better. My friend told her mum, and she told my mum. Mum was really upset but not angry – she said she was sad it had happened and that it wasn't my fault. She spoke to the police. A policewoman and social worker came to see me, they were really nice. They asked me to tell them what had happened – it took me a long time. It wasn't like on TV or anything, it was in a really ordinary room, not in a police station. They arrested my uncle.

We don't see my aunt now or my cousins because they are upset that mum spoke to the police. Mum says it's better that we did, that it's better it stopped and that we're safe. I feel a lot better now.' ✪

- be fearful and frightened of physical contact
- become depressed and take an overdose or harm themselves
- run away, become promiscuous or take to prostitution
- drink too much or start using drugs
- develop an eating disorder such as anorexia or bulimia.

Emotionally abused or neglected children may:

- be slow to learn to walk and talk
- be very passive and unable to be spontaneous
- have feeding problems and grow slowly
- find it hard to develop close relationships
- be over-friendly with strangers
- get on badly with other children of the same age
- be unable to play imaginatively
- think badly of themselves
- be easily distracted and do badly at school.

What can I do to help?

First and foremost, the child must be protected from further abuse. If you suspect that a child is being abused, you may be able to help them to talk about it.

Social Services will need to be involved to find out:

- what has happened
- whether it is likely to happen again
- what steps are needed to protect the child.

Your local Social Services child protection advisor will be able to offer more detailed information. It is helpful to speak to them even if you are not sure. Remember, all of us need to protect the child from further harm.

Child protection

After investigation, Social Services may be satisfied that the problems have been sorted out, and that the parents can now care for and protect the child properly. If so, they will remain involved only if the family wants their help. If Social Services are concerned that a child is being harmed, they will arrange a child protection case conference. The parents and professionals who know the child will be invited. A plan will be made to help the child and family and ensure that there is no further harm.

Help to look after the child

When a child has been abused within the family, the person involved is sometimes able to own up to what they have done and wants help. They can then be helped to look after their child better. Occasionally, the child may have to be taken away from the abusing adult because the risks of physical and emotional harm are too great. This can be for a short time, until things become safer, or may be permanent.

Specialist treatment

Many children need specialist treatment because of the abuse they have endured. Some receive help from **family centres** run by Social Services. If they are worried, depressed or being very difficult, the child and family might need help from the local child and adolescent mental health service (**CAMHS**). These specialists may work with the whole family or with children and adolescents alone. Sometimes they work with teenagers in groups. Individual therapy can be especially helpful for children who have been sexually abused, or who have experienced severe trauma. Children who have suffered serious abuse or neglect can be difficult to care for, and the service can offer help and advice to parents and carers.

Recommended reading

Other factsheets in this series: Traumatic stress in children, Domestic violence, CAMHS

The Young Mind: An Essential Guide to Mental Health for Young Adults, Parents and Teachers, edited by Sue Bailey and Mike Shooter (2009) – an accessible, user-friendly handbook produced by the Royal College of Psychiatrists.

References

Amaya-Jackson L. Understanding the behavioral and emotional consequences of child abuse. Committee on Child Abuse and Neglect and Section on Adoption and Foster Care. *Pediatrics* 2008; 122: 667–73.

Gilbert R, Spatz Widom C, Browne K, et al. Burden and consequences of child maltreatment in high income countries. *Lancet* 2009; 373: 68–81.

HM Government. *Working Together to Safeguard Children: A Guide to Inter-Agency Working to Safeguard and Promote the Welfare of Children*. Department for Children, Schools and Families, 2010.

Rutter M, Bishop D, Pine D, et al (eds) *Rutter's Child and Adolescent Psychiatry* (5th edn). Wiley–Blackwell, 2008.

Useful websites

- **ChildLine**: www.childline.org.uk; provides free and confidential service for children. Helpline: 0800 1111.
- **National Society for the Prevention of Cruelty to Children (NSPCC)**: www.nspcc.org.uk; NSPCC has a number of useful publications. If you are worried about a child, call their helpline: 0808 800 5000.
- **The Hideout**: www.thehideout.org.uk; a website offering support and advice to children whose lives are affected by domestic abuse.
- **Young Carers**: www.youngcarers.net; a website offering support, information and advice for children who also act as carers.
- **Barnardo's**: www.barnardos.org.uk; works with families and children in many ways, including counselling, fostering and adoption, support for young carers, training and disability inclusion.

Notes

19 Drugs and alcohol: what parents need to know
Information for parents, carers and anyone who works with young people

This is one in a series of factsheets for parents, teachers and anyone who works with young people, with practical, up-to-date information about mental health problems (emotional, behavioural and psychiatric disorders) that can affect children and young people.

This factsheet offers practical advice for parents, teachers and carers who are worried that a young person is misusing drugs or alcohol.

What are the different types of drugs which cause problems?

The most commonly used, readily available and strongly addictive drugs are **tobacco** and **alcohol**. There are numerous others that can be addictive.

Alcohol and **cannabis** are sometimes seen as 'gateway' drugs that lead to the world of other drugs like cocaine and heroin.

Drugs are also classed as 'legal' and 'illegal'. The obviously illegal drugs include cannabis (hash), speed (amphetamines), ecstasy (E), cocaine and heroin. Using 'legal' drugs (e.g. cigarettes, alcohol, petrol, glue) does not mean they are safe or allowed to be misused. It just means they may be bought or sold for specific purposes and are limited to use by specific age groups.

There are clear laws regarding alcohol and young people. For more detailed information on various drugs, their side-effects and the law, see 'Useful websites' at the end of this factsheet.

Why do young people use drugs or alcohol?

Young people may try or use drugs or alcohol for various reasons. They may do it for fun, because they are curious, or to be like their friends. Some are experimenting with the feeling of intoxication. Sometimes they use it to cope with difficult situations or feelings of worry and low mood. A young person is more likely to try or use drugs or alcohol if they hang out or stay with friends or family who use them.

Why do I need to know about a young person using drugs or alcohol?

Many young people smoke, drink alcohol and may try drugs. It is important you are aware of this and do not ignore it as a time when they are just having fun or experimenting. It does not take much for the young person to lose control and to need help to recover from this problem.

By the age of 16, up to half of young people have tried an illegal drug. Young people are trying drugs earlier and more are drinking alcohol.

What can be the problems related to using drugs or alcohol?

Drugs and alcohol can have different effects on different people. In young people especially the effects can be **unpredictable** and potentially **dangerous**. Even medications for sleep or painkillers can be addictive and harmful if not used the way they are prescribed by a doctor.

Drugs and alcohol can **damage health**. Sharing needles or equipment can cause serious infections, such as **HIV** and **hepatitis**. Accidents, arguments and **fights** are more likely after drinking and drug use. Young people are more likely to engage in **unprotected sex** when using drugs.

Using drugs can lead to **serious mental illnesses**, such as psychosis and depression.

When does it become a problem or addiction?

It is very difficult to know when exactly using drugs or alcohol is more than just 'casual'.

Addiction becomes more obvious when the young person spends most of their time thinking about, looking for or using drugs. Drugs or alcohol then become the focus of the young person's life. They ignore their usual work, for example schoolwork, or stop doing their usual hobbies/sports such as dancing or football.

How do I know if it becomes a problem or addiction?

Occasional use can be very difficult to detect. If the young person is using a drug on a regular basis, their behaviour often changes. Look for signs such as:

- unexplained moodiness
- behaviour that is 'out of character'
- loss of interest in school or friends
- unexplained loss of clothes or money
- unusual smells and items like silver foil or needle covers.

Remember, the above changes can also mean other problems, such as depression, rather than using drugs.

What do I do if I am worried?

If you suspect a young person is using drugs, remember some general rules.

- Pay attention to what the child is doing, including schoolwork, friends and leisure time.
- Learn about the effects of alcohol and drugs (websites listed at the end of this factsheet contain some useful information).
- Listen to what the child says about alcohol and drugs, and talk about it with them.
- Encourage the young person to be informed and responsible about drugs and alcohol.
- Talk to other parents, friends or teachers about drugs, the facts and your fears and **seek help**.

If someone in the family or a close friend is using drugs or alcohol, it is important that they seek help too. It may be hard to expect the young person to give up, especially if a parent or carer is using too.

My child is abusing drugs. What do I do?

- If your child is using drugs or alcohol, seek help.
- Stay calm and make sure of the acts.
- Don't give up on them and don't get into long debates or arguments when they are drunk, stoned or high.
- Don't be angry or blame them – they need your help and trust to recover.

Where can I get help?

You can talk in confidence to a professional such as your GP or practice nurse, a local drug project or your local child and adolescent mental health service (CAMHS). They can refer your child to relevant services and they will be able to offer you advice and support.

You may also be able to seek help through a school nurse, teacher or social worker. You can find this information from your local area telephone book or council website, or ask for the address from your health centre.

You may also look at the websites listed at the end of this factsheet. Most offer telephone advice and email contact.

Michelle, mum, talks about Johnny's drug use

'Johnny was always the boisterous one with a short fuse. So unlike his brother Jack and sister Lucy. He was good with doing things like making and fixing stuff, but not very good in English or other subjects. I thought he was more like his dad, Jake. Jake was away most of the time working as a truck driver. It was like being a single parent with three kids. I looked after the home, cooked, fed the kids and cleaned the house. But maybe I never spent much time with the kids. They were all good so I never really thought about it. Not until the day Jack came and told us about Johnny missing school and having bruises all over. I don't know how I missed it... there were some signs but I had just thought it was him being a teenager. Johnny's clothes were smelly, he used to come home really late at weekends and he did not look healthy.

He did not even eat much and only had coffee in the morning. It was like walking on fire when we first asked Johnny... I thought his life was over. I cried, felt guilty. The drug counsellor told us all about drugs, how we could help. Somehow I felt there was a ray of hope. It has been a long, rocky road but I feel stronger. Johnny is enjoying his vocational courses. We make sure we spend time as a family, go out, even though we can't afford much.

I wish I had known about these things before... maybe a parents' evening in school would've helped.' ✪

Recommended reading

Other factsheets in this series:

CAMHS

A Parent's Guide to Drugs and Alcohol, published by the Department of Health, 2006, is a useful guide containing basic information and links where to find help.

References

Chick J. *Understanding Alcohol and Drinking Problems. British Medical Association's Family Doctor Series.* BMA, 2006.

National Institute for Health and Clinical Excellence. *Drug Misuse: Opioid Detoxification* (CG52). NICE, 2007.

National Institute for Health and Clinical Excellence. *Drug Misuse: Psychosocial Interventions* (CG51). NICE, 2007.

National Institute for Health and Clinical Excellence. *Treating Harmful Drinking and Alcohol Dependence.* NICE, 2011 (www.nice.org.uk/nicemedia/live/13337/53199/53199.pdf)

Rutter M, Bishop D, Pine D, et al (eds) *Rutter's Child and Adolescent Psychiatry* (5th edn). Wiley–Blackwell, 2008.

Useful websites

- **Alcohol Concern**: www.alcoholconcern.org.uk; national agency campaigning for effective alcohol policy and improved services for people whose lives are affected by alcohol-related problems.
- **NHS Choices**: www.nhs.uk; website with health information and a section on alcohol and drugs.
- **Drink Sense**: www.drinksense.org; counselling, information and support for people with alcohol-related problems, their carers and families. Has information for young people under the age of 25.
- **Patient UK**: www.patient.co.uk; information on health issues, including alcohol and drug misuse and links to various useful books and websites.
- **NHS Direct**: www.nhsdirect.nhs.uk; help and advice on any aspect of drug and alcohol use. Tel: 0845 4647.
- **Smokefree**: http://smokefree.nhs.uk; NHS smoking helpline: 0800 022 4 332.
- **Talk to Frank**: www.talktofrank.com; free, confidential drugs information and advice line. Tel. 0800 77 66 00.
- **Addaction**: www.addaction.org.uk; specialist drug and alcohol treatment charity in England and Scotland.

Notes

....

....

....

....

....

....

....

....

20 Self-harm in young people
Information for parents, carers and anyone who works with young people

This is one in a series of factsheets for parents, teachers and anyone who works with young people, with practical, up-to-date information about mental health problems (emotional, behavioural and psychiatric disorders) that can affect children and young people.

This factsheet looks at the reasons behind why young people self-harm, and offers advice about what to do to help.

Why do young people harm themselves?

Some young people use self-harm as a way of trying to deal with very difficult feelings that build up inside them. This is clearly very serious and can be life-threatening. People say different things about why they do it.

- Some say that they have been feeling desperate about a problem and don't know where to turn for help. They feel trapped and helpless. Self-injury helps them to **feel more in control**.

- Some people talk of feelings of anger or tension that get bottled up inside, until they feel like exploding. Self-injury helps to **relieve the tension** that they feel.

- Feelings of guilt or shame may also become unbearable. Self-harm is way of **punishing oneself**.

- Some people try to cope with very upsetting experiences, such as trauma or abuse, by convincing themselves that the upsetting event(s) never happened. These people sometimes feel 'numb' or 'dead'. They say that they feel detached from the world and their bodies, and that self-injury is a way of **feeling more connected and alive**.

- A proportion of young people who self-harm do so because they feel so upset and overwhelmed that they wish to end their lives by **dying** by suicide. At the time, many people just want their problems to disappear, and have no idea how to get help. They feel as if the only way out is to kill themselves.

> ### What is self-harm?
> Self-harm is a term used when someone injures or harms themselves on purpose rather than by accident. Common examples include overdosing (self-poisoning), hitting, cutting or burning oneself, pulling hair or picking skin, or self-strangulation. Self-harm is always a sign of something being seriously wrong.

Who is at risk?

An episode of self-harm is most commonly triggered by an argument with a parent or close friend. When family life involves a lot of abuse, neglect or rejection, people are more likely to harm themselves. Young people who are depressed, or have an eating disorder, or another serious mental health problem, are more likely to self-harm. So are people who take illegal drugs or drink too much alcohol.

Many young people who self-harm with a wish to die by suicide also have mental health or personality difficulties; often the suicide attempt follows a stressful event in the young person's life, but in other cases, the young person may not have shown any previous signs of difficulty.

Sometimes the young person is known to have long-standing difficulties at school, home or with the police. Some will already be seeing a counsellor, psychiatrist or social worker. There has been an increase in the suicide rate in young men over recent years.

The risk of suicide is higher if the young person:

- is depressed, or has a serious mental illness
- is using drugs or alcohol when they are upset
- has previously tried to kill themselves, or has planned for a while about how to die without being saved
- has a relative or friend who tried to kill themselves.

How can I help?

- **Notice** when the young person seems upset, withdrawn or irritable. Self-injury is often kept secret but there may be clues, such as refusing to wear short sleeves or to take off clothing for sports.
- **Encourage** them to talk about their worries and take them seriously. Show them you care by listening, offer sympathy and understanding, and help them to solve any problems.
- **Buy blister packs of medicine in small amounts.** This helps prevent impulsive overdoses. Getting pills out of a blister pack takes longer than swallowing them straight from a bottle. It may be long enough to make someone stop and think about what they are doing.
- **Keep medicines locked away.**
- **Get help** if family problems or arguments keep upsetting you or the young person.
- If a young person has injured themselves, you can **help practically** by checking to see whether injuries (cuts or burns for example) need hospital treatment and if not, by providing them with clean dressings to cover their wounds.

As a parent, it is really hard to cope with a child/young person with self-harming behaviour or who attempts suicide. It is natural to feel angry, frightened or guilty. It may also be difficult to take it seriously or know what to do for the best. Try to keep calm and caring, even if you feel cross or frightened; this will show your child you can manage their distress and they can come to you for help and support.

This may be difficult if there are a lot of problems or arguments at home. Or, you may simply feel too upset, angry or overwhelmed to effectively help your child/young person. If so, you should seek advice from your GP.

If you are a teacher, it is important to encourage students to let you know if one of their friends is in trouble, upset or shows signs of harming themselves. Friends often worry about betraying a confidence and you may need to explain that self-harm is very serious and can be life-threatening. For this reason, it should never be kept secret.

Where do I get specialist help?

Everyone who has taken an overdose or tried to kill themselves needs an urgent assessment by a doctor as soon as possible, even if they look OK. Usually, this means an examination at the nearest emergency department (also known as A&E). If you are unsure whether the young person was suicidal or not, it is best to act cautiously and take them to hospital. With overdose, the harmful effects can sometimes be delayed, and treatment with medication may be needed. Paracetamol is the most common medicine taken as an overdose in Britain. It can cause serious liver damage, and each year this leads to many deaths. Even small overdoses can sometimes be fatal.

If the young person is self-harming by cutting themselves or in other ways, it is still important that they have help. Speak to your GP who can refer you to your local child and adolescent mental health services (CAMHS).

Michelle, 16

'I've always been the tallest girl in my class and my so-called friends regularly bitch about me behind my back and bully me. I hate being different, but the harder I try to fit in, the more they reject me.

My parents are divorced and I lived for many years with my mother but it was my grandmother who really looked after me. My mother was always busy at work or with her friends or boyfriend; she travelled a lot. I never felt that she was really there for me. My father remarried to a much younger woman who hated me and I hated her – I still do.

A couple of years ago, I was changing for PE and noticed that one of my friends had bright red lines all the way down her arms; she usually wore long-sleeved tops, even in the summer, so I had never noticed them before. I was shocked and she confided in me that she regularly cut herself. I couldn't understand why – she had everything, rich parents and wonderful holidays all over the world. She told me that her parents were never around and that she spent a lot of her time by herself. She felt that when she cut herself, she got rid of the pain and the loneliness.

I am now 16 and have been regularly cutting myself for more than a year. I hide the knife or the scissors under the mattress and when my mother goes to bed, I cut my arms and the top of my thighs. Some days are worse than others, particularly when I get upset.

My mother noticed the marks on my body and took me to the GP who put me on antidepressants, but I never took them. I am now seeing a psychotherapist. I go every week, but I still have a lot of things to sort out and it's taking time. I'm not doing it so often, only when I feel very stressed. I know it's dangerous, but it's a very difficult thing to stop doing.' ✪

How is self-harm treated?

- **Assessment**

  All young people who attend hospital following attempting suicide or harming themselves should also have a specialist mental health assessment before leaving.

  It is often difficult to work out what prompted the young person to self-harm or whether they actually wished to die by suicide or not; mental health professionals have the expertise to make sense of these complicated situations.

- **Parental involvement**

  It is usual for parents or carers to be involved in the assessment and any treatment. This makes it easier to understand the background to what has happened, and to work out together whether more help is needed.

  Assessments in emergency departments (A&E) which include a short 'talking therapy' session have been shown to help young people come back for ongoing help and support. A lot of young people self-harm or make another suicide attempt if they do not receive the help they need.

- **Therapy**

  Usually, treatment for self-harm and attempted suicide, other than any immediate physical treatment, will involve individual or family 'talking therapy' work for a small number of sessions. They will need help with how to cope with the very difficult feelings that cause self-harm.

- **Treatment plan**

  Clear plans on how to help and how to keep the young person safe will also be made. Some people who find it very difficult to stop self-harming behaviour in the short term will need help to think of less harmful ways of managing their distress.

  Families often need help in working out how to make sure that the dangerous behaviour does not happen again, and how to give the support that is needed. This is something your local CAMHS should have on offer.

- **Long-term specialist help**

  If depression or another serious mental health problem is part of the problem, it will need treatment. Some young people who self-harm may have suffered particularly damaging and traumatic experiences in their past. A very small number of young people who try to kill themselves really do still want to die. These two groups may need specialist help over a longer period of time.

Recommended reading

Other factsheets in this series: Traumatic stress in children, Divorce or separation of parents, Worries and anxieties, The emotional cost of bullying, CAMHS

Changing Minds. Mental Health: What it is, What to do, Where to go? This is a CD produced by the Royal College of Psychiatrists for 13- to 17-year-olds. It talks about addiction, stress, eating disorders, depression, schizophrenia and self-harm.

The Young Mind: An Essential Guide to Mental Health for Young Adults, Parents and Teachers, edited by Sue Bailey and Mike Shooter (2009) – an accessible, user-friendly handbook produced by the Royal College of Psychiatrists.

Understanding NICE Guidance. There are versions of all guidance for patients, carers and the public and summarises, in plain English, the recommendations that the National Institute for Health and Clinical Excellence makes to health and other professionals.

References

Hawton K, Harriss L. Deliberate self-harm in young people: characteristics and subsequent mortality in a 20-year cohort of patients presenting to hospital. *J Clin Psychiatry* 2007; 68: 1574–83.

National Institute for Health and Clinical Excellence. *Longer-Term Care and Treatment of Self-Harm.* NICE, 2011.

National Institute for Health and Clinical Excellence. *Self-Harm: The Short-Term Physical and Psychological Management of Secondary Prevention of Self-Harm in Primary and Secondary Care* (CG16). NICE, 2004.

Ougrin D, Zundel T, Ng A, et al. Trial of Therapeutic Assessment in London: randomised controlled trial of Therapeutic Assessment versus standard psychosocial assessment in adolescents presenting with self-harm. *Arch Dis Child* 2011; 96: 148–53.

Useful websites

➲ **National Self Harm Network**: www.nshn.co.uk; UK charity offering support, advice and advocacy services to people affected by self-harm directly or in a care role.

➲ **ChildLine**: www.childline.org.uk; provides a free and confidential telephone service for children. Helpline: 0800 1111.

➲ **YoungMinds**: www.youngminds.org.uk; provides information and advice on child mental health issues and a parents' helpline: 0808 802 5544

➲ **The Samaritans**: www.samaritans.org.uk; a 24-hour service offering confidential emotional support to anyone who is in crisis. Helpline: 08457 909090 (UK), 1850 609090 (Northern Ireland), email: jo@ samaritans.org

➲ **Life Signs**: www.lifesigns.org.uk; an online, user-led voluntary organisation to raise awareness about self-injury and provide information and support to people of all ages affected by self-injury.

➲ **NHS Direct**: www.nhsdirect.nhs.uk; health advice and information service. Tel: 0845 4647

Notes

For a catalogue of public education materials or copies of our leaflets contact: Book Sales/Leaflets, The Royal College of Psychiatrists, 17 Belgrave Square, London SW1X 8PG. Email: leaflets@rcpsych.ac.uk, tel: 020 7235 2351 ext. 6146.

Revised by the Royal College of Psychiatrists' Child and Family Public Education Editorial Board. With grateful thanks to Dr Vasu Balaguru and Dr Mona Freeman. This leaflet reflects the best possible evidence at the time of writing.

21 Psychosis
Information for parents, carers and anyone who works with young people

This is one in a series of factsheets for parents, teachers and anyone who works with young people, with practical, up-to-date information about mental health problems (emotional, behavioural and psychiatric disorders) that can affect children and young people.

This factsheet explains what psychosis is and gives practical help and advice about how and where to get help for young people affected by this mental illness.

How common is it?

'Psychosis' can affect people of all ages, but becomes increasingly common as people reach young adulthood.

What causes psychosis?

When a person has a psychotic episode, it can be a signal of an underlying illness. You can have a 'psychotic breakdown' after a stressful event such as losing a close friend or relative. It can also be the result of a physical illness like a severe infection, the use of illegal drugs like cannabis, or a severe mental illness like schizophrenia or bipolar disorder. Sometimes it is difficult to know what caused the illness.

> ### What is psychosis?
> The term 'psychosis' is used to describe a situation when a person loses touch with reality. Young people can behave very differently when they are feeling stressed, confused or very upset. In fact, these are rarely signs of mental illness. Psychosis is usually more severe and disabling.

What are the symptoms of psychosis?

When a person has psychosis, they may have unusual thoughts and experiences. These may appear suddenly, or develop gradually over time. People may have one or more of the symptoms.

- **Unusual beliefs called delusions.** These unshakeable beliefs are obviously untrue to others, but may not be so to the young person themselves. For example, when a young person is ill, they may think that there is a plot to harm them, or that they are being spied on by the TV, or being taken over by aliens. Sometimes they may feel they are a special person or have special powers.
- **Thought disorder** is when they are not able to think straight. It may be difficult to understand what they are saying; their ideas may seem jumbled, but it is more than being muddled or confused.
- **Unusual experiences called hallucinations** are when they can see, hear, smell or feel something that isn't really there. The most common hallucination people experience is hearing voices. In psychosis, hallucinations are totally real to the person having them. This can be very frightening and can make them believe that they are being watched or picked on.

Having these strange thoughts and experiences can affect a young person at school, at home or when with friends. They may find it difficult to concentrate and enjoy what they normally did. It can even affect their sleep, appetite and physical health.

How to get help

The earlier it is recognised that a young person is ill, the better the chances of getting effective treatment. This speeds recovery and reduces long-term harm. Some people can make a complete recovery.

Even if your child won't come with you, it is helpful to speak to your GP. It is likely that they will be referred to a psychiatrist in a child and adolescent mental health service (CAMHS) or an early intervention team or service, if this is available locally. Early intervention teams are specialists in dealing with young people with psychosis. If your child is very unwell, they may need admission to hospital until their condition stabilises.

What is the treatment for psychosis?

- Medical treatment

  Medications called **antipsychotics** are an important part of treatment. They may need to be taken for a long time for the child to stay well. As with medication of any kind, there may be side-effects; the psychiatrist will be able to advise on what they are and what can be done to help. The risk of side-

Luke, 16, talks about psychosis

'I was about 14 when it happened. I had a good family, did well at school and had a group of good friends. Life had been good to me, although my mum said I could not handle stress. I would be a bag of nerves before exams, was scared of failing and could not face it if someone was unwell.

Uncle Rob's death a year back in the accident was just too much. I knew I would feel upset for a long time. But then I didn't feel upset. It was strange. I thought people were doing strange things to me like controlling me through radio signals. I felt I had lost control of myself and even felt my body was changing in a strange sort of way. And then I could not face school, I was swearing, felt muddled in my head. My learning mentor got worried and spoke to my mum, who had noticed my strange behaviour. I couldn't sleep and couldn't be bothered about going out. I didn't like the idea of seeing a psychiatrist from the child and adolescent mental health service and I thought they would judge me. But it was very different. She seemed to know and understand how I felt, what I thought. I felt relieved. She even said I was not going to be locked away in a hospital. It was just an illness for which I needed to take medication for a few months or a year. She then introduced me to Kay, a worker from an early intervention psychosis team. Kay explained to me and my family all about psychosis, what we could do to keep me well. She was there when I felt I was losing it before my exams.

It's nearly 2 years now. I am like any other 16-year-old, going to school, meeting with friends, etcetera. I take my meds and stay away from drugs and alcohol.' ✪

effects needs to be balanced against the risk of the damaging effects of the illness on a young person's life.

Some of the medicines for the treatment of psychosis are unlicensed for children and young people. This does not mean they do not work for young people, but simply that the drug company has not applied for a licence. If you are worried about this, you should speak to the doctor or pharmacist. Further information is also available from the Royal College of Paediatrics and Child Health.

If the psychosis is related to drug use or underlying physical problems, your child may need specific help and treatment to manage this.

- **Therapy**

  Other forms of treatment in addition to medicine are also important. **Talking treatments** can be helpful. The whole family will need help to understand more about the illness, to cope successfully, and to help prevent the illness coming back.

What will happen in the future?

With early help and treatment, most young people recover from their psychotic episode. If the illness is due to an underlying physical illness or using drugs, they may be able to avoid having another episode by taking appropriate treatment and avoiding taking drugs.

When a young person has a psychotic breakdown that has not been caused by drug use, it can be difficult to know what the long-term effects will be and a definite diagnosis may not be possible straight away. Some young people may eventually be diagnosed with a severe mental illness like schizophrenia or bipolar disorder.

Is there anything else I should do?

You can help as a parent by supporting your child to continue with any treatment offered and to keep a balanced, healthy lifestyle. You may be able to identify the signs early if their illness recurs in the future, and seek help more quickly.

Recommended reading

Other factsheets in this series: Schizophrenia, Bipolar disorder, CAMHS

References

National Institute for Health and Clinical Excellence. *Core Interventions in the Treatment and Management of Schizophrenia in Primary and Secondary Care* (update) (CG82). NICE, 2009.

Rutter M, Bishop D, Pine D, et al (eds) *Rutter's Child and Adolescent Psychiatry* (5th edn). Wiley–Blackwell, 2008.

Useful websites

- ⊃ **Mind**: www.mind.org.uk; national mental health charity for England and Wales.

- ⊃ **TalktoFrank**: www.talktofrank.com; has information on drug use and drug-induced psychosis.

- ⊃ **Young Minds**: www.youngminds.org.uk; a charity that offers information to young people about mental health and emotional well-being.

22 Schizophrenia
Information for parents, carers and anyone who works with young people

This is one in a series of factsheets for parents, teachers and anyone who works with young people, with practical, up-to-date information about mental health problems (emotional, behavioural and psychiatric disorders) that can affect children and young people.

This factsheet explains what schizophrenia is and gives practical help and advice about how and where to get help for young people affected by this mental illness.

What are the symptoms of schizophrenia?

Schizophrenia affects everybody differently. There are two groups of symptoms, which are described as 'positive' and 'negative'. This doesn't mean that some are good and some are bad; more that some are about 'doing' things or experiencing symptoms, and some are about 'not doing' things. Young people with schizophrenia often have a mixture of the two.

Sometimes, the illness develops slowly and can be hard to spot, whereas in other young people the illness begins very quickly.

Positive symptoms

- **Strange beliefs or delusions** are very strongly held beliefs that are not only untrue, but can seem quite bizarre. The young person may believe that they are someone different, a world leader or celebrity for example, or they may believe that other people are 'out to get them'. They will believe this is true, no matter what you say.
- **Thought disorder** is when someone is not thinking straight and it is hard to make sense of what they are saying. Their ideas may be jumbled up, but it is more than being muddled or confused.
- **Hallucinations** are when someone sees, hears, smells or feels something that isn't really there. The most common hallucination that people have is hearing voices. In schizophrenia, hallucinations are totally real to the person having them. This can be very frightening and can make them believe that they are being watched or picked on. People who are having these experiences may act strangely. For example, they may talk or laugh to themselves, or appear to be talking to somebody that others can't see.

What is schizophrenia?

Schizophrenia is a serious mental illness that affects thinking, emotions and behaviour. It is the most common form of psychosis.

Over a lifetime, about 1 in 100 people will develop schizophrenia. It is most likely to start between the ages of 15 and 35, but can sometimes occur in younger children. The illness might last for a long time and can be very disabling.

Negative symptoms

The young person who has schizophrenia can become **withdrawn** and appear **unemotional**. They seem to lose interest, stop washing regularly and can spend a lot of time on their own. They may not be able to carry on with their normal activities, and usually find it **difficult to concentrate** on work or study.

Other symptoms

Some young people can become **frustrated** and **angry**, even towards their own family. Others may take drugs or drink alcohol to feel better. Some find the symptoms so distressing that they want to **self-harm**.

In spite of how they are described in the media, people who have schizophrenia are not more dangerous or violent than anyone else. However, they may come across as worrying and unpredictable, especially when they feel **frightened** by their strange experiences.

What causes schizophrenia?

We do not know the exact cause of schizophrenia, although it does seem to relate to chemical imbalances in the brain. Research shows that having parents or close relatives with mental illness, experiencing stress and using drugs, such as cannabis, can all be associated with having schizophrenia.

How do I get help?

The earlier it is recognised that a young person is ill, the better the chances of getting effective treatment. This speeds recovery and reduces the long-term harm. Some people can make a complete recovery.

Even if your child won't come with you, you might find it helpful to talk to your GP. It is likely that they will be referred to a psychiatrist in a child and adolescent mental health service (CAMHS) or an early intervention team or service (EIS) if this is available locally. Professionals from the early intervention team are specialists in working with young people with psychosis. If your child is very unwell, they may need admission to hospital for a period of time until their condition stabilises.

What is the treatment for schizophrenia?

Medications called **antipsychotics** are an important part of the treatment of schizophrenia. They treat the symptoms of the illness, but tend to be more effective with positive symptoms than negative symptoms. Hallucinations and delusions may take weeks and sometimes months to improve. Unfortunately, schizophrenia can recur, and may need long-term treatment.

A number of different antipsychotics are available, and the psychiatrist will advise which is the best for your child. Sometimes, several different drugs will need to be tried to find the most effective one.

As with all medication, there can be **side-effects**. The psychiatrists will advise on these and what can be done to help. The risk of side-effects needs to be balanced against the risk of the damaging effects of the illness on a young person's life.

Some medicines for the treatment of schizophrenia are unlicensed for children and young people. This does not mean they do not work, but simply that the drug company has not applied for a licence. If you are worried about this, you should speak to your doctor or pharmacist.

Practical help and support

It is crucial that medication is combined with practical help and support for the young person and their family. This should cover several aspects.

- **Understanding the illness**
  It is very important that the young person with schizophrenia and their family are helped to understand the condition.

- **Resuming education, training or starting work**
  An episode of schizophrenia can interfere with education because it is difficult for a young person to learn when unwell. An important part of recovery is to plan for their future.

- **Family relationships**
  Experiencing stress, hostility and criticism can all increase the chance of relapse. Families need help with recognising and reducing these factors, and with how best to support the young person. Young people with schizophrenia can live independently just like peers of their own age. Their family and professionals working with them may need to support and help them in this process.

- **Coping with specific symptoms**
  Some people with schizophrenia find cognitive–behavioural therapy (CBT) helpful in managing hallucinations, in addition to the medicine prescribed.

Recommended reading

Other factsheets in this series:
CAMHS

Surviving Schizophrenia: A Manual for Families, Patients and Providers, by E. Fuller-Torrey. Quill, 2006.

The Young Mind: An Essential Guide to Mental Health for Young Adults, Parents and Teachers, edited by Sue Bailey and Mike Shooter (2009) – an accessible, user-friendly handbook produced by the Royal College of Psychiatrists.

References

National Institute for Health and Clinical Health and Excellence. *Core Interventions in the Treatment and Management of Schizophrenia in Primary and Secondary Care* (update) (CG82). NICE, 2009.

Rutter M, Bishop D, Pine D, et al (eds) *Rutter's Child and Adolescent Psychiatry* (5th edn). Wiley–Blackwell, 2008.

Useful websites

- **Mind**: www.mind.org.uk; a national mental health charity for England and Wales.
- **Young Minds**: www.youngminds.org.uk; for any adult concerned about the emotions and behaviour of a child or young person. Parents' helpline: 0808 802 5544.
- **TalktoFrank**: www.talktofrank.com; information on drugs and drug-induced psychosis.

Notes

....

....

....

....

....

....

....

....

....

....

23 Bipolar disorder in children and adolescents
Information for parents, carers and anyone who works with young people

This is one in a series of factsheets for parents, teachers and anyone who works with young people, with practical, up-to-date information about mental health problems (emotional, behavioural and psychiatric disorders) that can affect children and young people.

This factsheet gives some basic information about the symptoms and effects of bipolar disorder, and gives some practical advice on how to get help for this problem.

How common is bipolar disorder?

Bipolar disorder is extremely rare before puberty but becomes slightly more common during teenage years. It occurs in 1 in 100 or fewer children and teenagers. In adults it affects 1 in 100 people.

The condition can be hard to recognise in teenagers because more extreme behaviour can be part of this stage of life.

What causes it?

Although the causes are not fully understood, bipolar disorder tends to run in families. In people who have bipolar disorder, episodes may be triggered by physical illness, stressful events or lack of sleep.

What are the symptoms?

In bipolar disorder, a person can have:

- manic or hypomanic periods (or 'episodes') also known as 'highs'
- depressive periods also known as 'lows'
- mixed periods.

Below is a list of the symptoms in each episode. A young person needs to have at least one manic or hypomanic episode to be diagnosed with bipolar disorder. There needs to be several of these symptoms happening at the same time for at least several days. If there is just one symptom, then it is unlikely to be bipolar disorder.

The mood changes can sometimes occur very rapidly within hours or days ('rapid cycling'). For some, the mood symptoms are less severe ('cyclothymia').

In between the highs and lows, there are 'normal' periods that can last for weeks or months. However, for some, especially when they have had the disorder from some time, these periods of 'normalcy' can be shorter or difficult to see.

Symptoms during a 'high' or manic episode

- Feeling incredibly happy or 'high' in mood, uncontrolled excitement
- Irritability
- Increased talkativeness
- Very rapid speech with lots of changes of subject
- Racing thoughts
- Increased activity and restlessness
- Difficulty in concentrating or being easily distracted, constant changes in plans
- Overconfidence and inflated ideas about themselves or their abilities
- Needing little sleep
- Neglect of personal care
- Increased sociability or overfamiliarity
- Increased sexual energy
- Overspending of money or other types of reckless or extreme behaviour.

What is bipolar disorder?

Bipolar disorder is a condition in which a person has extreme changes of mood – periods of being unusually happy (known as 'mania' or 'hypomania'), and periods of being unusually sad ('depression'). It is sometimes called manic depressive disorder, bipolar affective disorder or bipolar mood disorder.

The mood swings are way beyond what would be considered normal for a particular individual, and are out of keeping with their personality.

'Hypomania' is a milder form of mania (less severe and for shorter periods). During these periods, people can actually become very productive and creative and so see these experiences as positive and valuable. However, hypomania, if left untreated, can become more severe, and may be followed by an episode of depression.

At the extreme end, some people also develop a condition called psychosis. This is when someone has strong, bizarre beliefs, for example that they have superhuman powers or are being watched or followed.

Symptoms during a 'low' or depressive episode

- Feeling very sad
- Decreased energy and activity
- Not being able to enjoy anything
- Decreased appetite
- Disturbed sleep
- Thoughts of suicide or self-harm.

On the milder end, one may just feel sad and gloomy all the time. Here, too, at the extreme end, some people can develop psychotic symptoms.

Symptoms during mixed episodes

A mixture of manic symptoms and depressive symptoms at the same time.

What effects can it have?

The exaggeration of thoughts, feelings and behaviour affects many areas of the young person's life. For example, it can lead to:

- problems in relationships with friends and family
- interference with concentration at school or work
- behaviour that places the young person's health or life at risk
- a loss of confidence and a loss of the sense of control over their life.

The longer the condition continues without treatment, the more harmful it is likely to be to the life of the young person and to their family.

Where can I get help?

The first step towards getting help is to recognise that there might be a problem. Seeking medical advice early on is very important. If the bipolar illness can be identified and treated quickly, this reduces its harmful effects.

You should contact your GP first. If necessary, they can then make a referral to your local child and adolescent mental health service (CAMHS) which can offer more specialist help.

How is it treated?

The goal of treatment is to improve the symptoms, prevent the illness from returning and help the young person lead a normal life. Families play an important role in preventing the illness from coming back, and also seeking help early before it becomes severe. It is therefore very important that you understand the condition.

Depending on whether the child is having a manic or a depressive episode and how severe it is, they may need different treatments. When they have severe symptoms they may need medications, and also sometimes admission to hospital.

Psychological or talking treatments and medication both may have an important role in the treatment of bipolar disorder.

> **Christina, 16**
>
> 'I was a happy, confident person studying for 11 GCSEs, and enjoying a good social life with a large circle of friends. All seemed well in my life. Suddenly, from feeling really cheerful, happy and full of energy, I withdrew to my room, stopped eating and stopped talking to everybody, even my parents. I was having vivid hallucinations, became paranoid and even thought about hurting myself.
>
> My parents became really worried and eventually I was admitted to a child and adolescent psychiatric unit. I now realise that I had mania before I plunged into black depression. Once I was diagnosed with bipolar disorder, I was able to understand and come to terms with my illness. Medication was given to me to deal with the mood swings, together with a talking therapy.
>
> With support from my family and friends, I am now back at school and I hope to go to medical school in the next couple of years.' ✪

Medication

Medication usually plays an important role in the treatment of bipolar disorder, especially if episodes are severe. In the initial stages of the illness, medication helps to reduce the symptoms.

The choice of medication can depend on the type of episode (manic or depressed). Everyone is different and so the type of medication that is recommended will also be different.

The three main types of medication that are helpful are:

- **antipsychotics:** risperidone, olanzapine and aripiprazole are types of antipsychotics
- **mood stabilisers:** lithium is a type of mood stabiliser
- **antidepressants:** fluoxetine is a type of antidepressant.

It is important that medications are not taken only when the problems are serious. If your child has had more than one severe episode of illness, staying on medication is important to reduce the risk of further episodes.

Medication may be needed for months or even years. Some people may, under medical supervision, be able to stop their medication when they have recovered and have felt well for a while. They may need physical examinations and tests (e.g. blood test) before starting or while on medication. It is important that if prescribed medication, the young person is regularly seen by their doctor or psychiatrist.

Side-effects of the medication can occur, some of which are quite serious. The psychiatrist will be able to advise about what they are and about what can be done to help. The risk of side-effects needs to be balanced against the risk of the damaging effects of the illness on a person's life.

No young person should be taking medication unless they are reviewed by a health professional regularly. This is to monitor the dose of the drug and to check for side-effects.

Talking treatments (also known as 'psychotherapies')

It is crucial that drug treatments are combined with practical help for the young person and their family.

- **Help with understanding the illness (psychoeducation)**

  It is very important that the young person with bipolar disorder and their family are helped to understand the condition, how best to cope and what to do to reduce the chances of it recurring.

  The young person and their family may notice particular 'triggers' to their episodes and/or early warning signs that an episode may be starting. Being aware of these can help reduce the chance of episodes occurring, and getting help in the earliest stages of an episode can stop it from escalating.

- **Family-focused treatment**

  Stress at home can worsen the situation and can even trigger an episode of the illness. Talking therapy in which the whole family is helped to find ways of reducing stress, solving problems and communicating more effectively has been shown to help young people with bipolar disorder get better, and stay well.

- **Cognitive–behavioural therapy (CBT)**

  This is another type of talking therapy in which the young person, sometimes with their family, learns to understand the links between their feelings and thoughts and how this affects their behaviour.

Hospital care

Some young people may need to go into hospital for intensive support if the symptoms are severe.

Rachel, 15

Rachel has suffered episodes of depression in the past. Two months ago she started to talk very quickly and seemed to have lots of energy. She was excited about everything and was making all her friends laugh a lot.

Over a 3-day period Rachel barely slept or ate and started to say things that did not really make sense; for example, she told friends that she was a princess in Taiwan. She also started swearing and became extremely flirtatious, which was out of character. She is quoted as saying, 'I've never felt so great – I'm flying. I'm eleven on a scale of one to ten.'

Rachel's parents were very worried and on the fourth night of her not sleeping, they took her to the local A&E department, where she was seen by a psychiatrist who arranged for her to stay in hospital. A diagnosis of bipolar disorder was confirmed and treatment was given to bring Rachel's mood back to normal. She now has treatment to help prevent episodes of both depressed and abnormally high mood in the future.

She has been working with a community psychiatric nurse to improve her ability to recognise her own mood state and take measures to protect herself from further episodes. ✪

Extract from The Young Mind: An Essential Guide to Mental Health for Young Adults, Parents and Teachers.

Recovery

It is important for the young person to recognise that they are not alone and to keep up hope.

Many people only have a few mood swings and then the problem goes away. For others, it becomes a lifelong pattern which they learn to live with and manage.

An episode of bipolar disorder can interfere with the young person's education because it is difficult to learn when they are unwell. An important part of recovery is to begin to plan returning to education or to think about work.

Useful websites

- **Bipolar UK**: www.bipolaruk.org.uk; supports people with a diagnosis of bipolar disorder and their families.
- **YoungMinds**: www.youngminds.org.uk; provides information and advice on child mental health issues. Parents' helpline: 0808 802 5544.
- **Rethink Mental Illness**: www.rethink.org; a national charity that helps people affected by a severe mental illness to recover a better quality of life.
- **SANE**: www.sane.org.uk; a national charity which improves the quality of life for people affected by mental illness.

Notes

....

....

....

....

....

....

....

....

....

....

....

....

....

Recommended reading

Other factsheets in this series: CBT (for young people), Psychosis, CAMHS

The Management of Bipolar Disorder in Adults, Children and Adolescents, in Primary and Secondary Care (CG38, patient version). National Institute for Health and Clinical Excellence, 2006.

The Young Mind: An Essential Guide to Mental Health for Young Adults, Parents and Teachers, edited by Sue Bailey and Mike Shooter (2009) – an accessible, user-friendly handbook produced by the Royal College of Psychiatrists.

References

Carr A. Bipolar disorder in young people: description, assessment and evidence-based treatment. *Dev Neurorehabil* 2009; 12; 427–41.

Fristad MA. Psychoeducational treatment for school-aged children with bipolar disorder. *Dev Psychopathol* 2006; 18: 1289–306.

Fristad MA, Verducci JS, Walters K, et al. Impact of multifamily psychoeducational psychotherapy in treating children aged 8 to 12 years with mood disorders. *Arch Gen Psychiatry* 2009; 66: 1013–21.

Leibenluft E, Dickstein DP. Bipolar disorder in children and adolescents. In *Rutter's Child and Adolescent Psychiatry* (5th edn) (eds M Rutter, D Bishop, D Pine, et al): 894–905. Wiley–Blackwell, 2008.

Merikangas KR, Akiskal HS, Angst J, et al. Lifetime and 12-month prevalence of bipolar spectrum disorder in the National Comorbidity Survey replication. *Arch Gen Psychiatry* 2007; 64: 543–52.

Miklowitz DJ, Axelson DA, Birmaher B, et al. Family-focused treatment for adolescents with bipolar disorder: results of a 2-year randomized trial. *Arch Gen Psychiatry* 2008; 65: 1053–61.

For a catalogue of public education materials or copies of our leaflets contact: Book Sales/Leaflets, The Royal College of Psychiatrists, 17 Belgrave Square, London SW1X 8PG. Email: leaflets@rcpsych.ac.uk, tel: 020 7235 2351 ext. 6146.

Revised by the Royal College of Psychiatrists' Child and Family Public Education Editorial Board. With grateful thanks to Dr Sarah Bates. This leaflet reflects the best possible evidence at the time of writing.

The Royal College of Psychiatrists is a charity registered in England and Wales (228636) and in Scotland (SC038369). © The Royal College of Psychiatrists 2013

24 Obsessive–compulsive disorder in children and young people
Information for parents, carers and anyone who works with young people

This is one in a series of factsheets for parents, teachers and anyone who works with young people, with practical, up-to-date information about mental health problems (emotional, behavioural and psychiatric disorders) that can affect children and young people.

This factsheet explains what obsessive–compulsive disorder is, who it affects and what can be done to help.

What are the symptoms of OCD?

Some people have thoughts, ideas or pictures that come into their mind over and over again. They are difficult to get rid of and can feel silly or unpleasant. These are called **obsessions**. Some examples of obsessions include:

- 'I must count to 20 or something bad will happen'
- worrying about germs and disease
- worrying about things being tidy.

Some people feel they have to do something repeatedly, even if they don't want to or it doesn't make sense. These are called **compulsions**. Some examples of compulsions include:

- repeatedly checking that the light is switched off
- washing hands again and again
- counting or repeating words in your head.

Often people try to stop themselves from doing these things, but feel frustrated or worried unless they can finish them. Problems with obsessions and compulsions can cause distress and worry, and can begin to affect young people at home with their families or at school with friends.

Many young people have mild obsessions and compulsions at some time, for example having to organise their toys in a special way, or saying good night a certain number of times. This is normal and may be the result of worry due to stress or change.

> ### What is obsessive–compulsive disorder (OCD)?
>
> The word 'obsessive' gets used commonly. This can mean different things to different people. Obsessive–compulsive disorder is a type of anxiety disorder. In this condition, the young person has obsessions and/or compulsions that affect their everyday life, for example getting to school on time, finishing homework or going out with friends.

How do I know this is OCD?

If you are worried that a young person may have OCD, you need to first think about these questions:

- Do the compulsions upset the child?
- Do they interfere with the child's everyday life (e.g. school, friends)?

If the answer to these questions is 'yes', it may be that the young person has OCD. If this is the case, you should seek professional advice.

How common is it?

Obsessive–compulsive disorder can affect people of all ages irrespective of their gender, religion or class. It usually starts in childhood. It is thought that 1–2% of the population have OCD, which means that at least 130 000 young people have it.

What causes OCD?

We do not know the cause of OCD for certain. Research suggests it may be due to an imbalance in a brain chemical called serotonin. It may also run in families and in people with tics (jerky movements). Very occasionally, OCD can start after an illness. It can also occur after a difficult time in a person's life, for example after having an accident.

How is OCD treated?

There are two treatments that are helpful for OCD: behaviour therapy and medication. These can be given on their own or together. If possible, a young person should have access to both forms of treatment.

- **Behaviour therapy**

  It starts with an assessment of the problem. This can include the young person and family keeping a diary of the obsessions and compulsions. The aim of the treatment is to teach the young person how to be in control of the problem, by tackling it a little bit at a time. The young person designs the treatment programme with the therapist as it is important to be actively involved in planning. Unless the condition is very severe, the most commonly used type of therapy is cognitive–behavioural therapy (CBT).

- **Exposure and response prevention (ERP)**

  This is when the therapist helps the child to face the things that they fear and have been avoiding. They are taught a wide range of skills to manage the anxiety that OCD creates.

  Often parents or other family members get very involved in the OCD rituals. Families need to learn about OCD, and also about how to help their child combat it. This can involve parents working with the child and therapist to find ways of helping their child to resist the rituals and being able to say 'no'.

- **Medication**

  Medication can be helpful in controlling the OCD. Unfortunately, many people who improve on medication become unwell again when the medication is stopped. Some people who need medication may have to continue taking it for a long time.

Where can I get help?

Obsessive–compulsive disorder is a common problem, and your GP will be able to help and advise you as to what you need to do. If the young person needs more specialist assessment and treatment, the GP may suggest a referral to a child and adolescent mental health service (CAMHS).

If the young person has been unwell for a long time, or their life has become severely affected by OCD, other professionals may need to help too; for example, teachers or educational social workers may be able to help the young person get back to ordinary life at school or college.

John, 18, talks about his OCD

'It started without me really noticing it. I got anxious about someone in my family dying – so I began to tap three times, when I got worried, for good luck and that would calm me down. Then I had to do it before I could go to sleep at night – not once but 3 x 3.

When I watched the programme on TV about those germs in hospital it began to get worse. I couldn't tell my mum or dad about it because it sounded so silly. I had to wash my hands all the time because I thought I would pass on an infection and someone would die. It was mainly at home, but then I began to worry that I would catch something at school.

I made my mum wash my school uniform every day. She tried to say no, but I would get so worked up that she would give in. It came to a head when I couldn't get to school on time because I was spending hours in the bathroom in the morning. I had to wash my hair three times as well as going through washing in a set order. If I was interrupted because someone needed the bathroom, I had to start again.

Mum got me some help. I didn't want to be seen as some psycho person, but Dr Roberts was really nice and understood why I was so worked up about everything. That was when I was 14. Now I am 18. It was hard work doing the therapy. It is called CBT. You have to try and work out why you are so anxious and try and control it. Now I am at college and doing a course that I like. I still do some counting, but I can keep it under control.' ✪

Recommended reading

Other factsheets in this series:
CBT (for young people), CAMHS

The Young Mind: An Essential Guide to Mental Health for Young Adults, Parents and Teachers, edited by Sue Bailey and Mike Shooter (2009) – an accessible, user-friendly handbook produced by the Royal College of Psychiatrists.

References

Heyman I. Children with obsessive–compulsive disorder. *BMJ* 1997; 315: 444.

National Institute for Health and Clinical Excellence. *Core Interventions in the Treatment of Obsessive–Compulsive Disorder and Body Dysmorphic Disorder* (CG31). NICE, 2005.

Office for National Statistics. *2011 Census for England and Wales*. ONS, 2011 (http://www.ons.gov.uk/ons/guide-method/census/2011/index.html).

Rutter M, Bishop D, Pine D, et al (eds) *Rutter's Child and Adolescent Psychiatry* (5th edn). Wiley–Blackwell, 2008.

Useful websites

- ⟳ **OCD Action**: www.ocdaction.org.uk; national charity for people with OCD and related disorders such as body dysmorphic disorder, compulsive skin picking and trichotillomania. Helpline: 0845 390 6232.

- ⟳ **International OCD Foundation**: www.ocfoundation.org; an international not-for-profit organisation made up of people who have OCD and related disorders, as well as their families, friends, professionals and others.

- ⟳ **OCD-UK**: www.ocduk.org; a national charity working with and for people with OCD.

Notes

....

....

....

....

....

....

....

....

For a catalogue of public education materials or copies of our leaflets contact: Book Sales/Leaflets, The Royal College of Psychiatrists, 17 Belgrave Square, London SW1X 8PG. Email: leaflets@rcpsych.ac.uk, tel: 020 7235 2351 ext. 6146.

Revised by the Royal College of Psychiatrists' Child and Family Public Education Editorial Board. With grateful thanks to Dr Kashmeera Naidoo. This leaflet reflects the best possible evidence at the time of writing.

25 Eating disorders in young people
Information for parents, carers and anyone who works with young people

This is one in a series of factsheets for parents, teachers and anyone who works with young people, with practical, up-to-date information about mental health problems (emotional, behavioural and psychiatric disorders) that can affect children and young people.

This factsheet discusses the causes of eating disorders and how to recognise them, as well as giving advice on how to cope with a child who has an eating disorder.

What are the signs of anorexia or bulimia?

You may notice some or most of these signs:

- weight loss or unusual weight changes
- periods being irregular or stopping
- missing meals, eating very little and avoiding 'fattening' foods
- avoiding eating in public, secret eating
- large amounts of food disappearing from the cupboards
- the person believing they are fat when in fact they are underweight
- exercising excessively, often in secret
- becoming preoccupied with food, cooking for other people, calorie counting and setting target weights
- going to the bathroom or toilet immediately after meals
- using laxatives and vomiting to control weight or sometimes using other medications/herbal remedies to lose weight.

It may be difficult for parents or teachers to tell the difference between ordinary dieting in young people and a more serious problem. If you are concerned about your child's weight and how they are eating, consult your GP. You can also seek help and advice from other agencies.

What effects can eating disorders have?

A person with an eating disorder can have physical and emotional problems. Some of these include:

- feeling excessively cold
- headaches and dizziness
- changes in hair and skin
- tiredness and difficulty with normal activities
- damage to health, including stunting of growth and damage to bones and internal organs
- loss of periods and risk of infertility
- anxiety and depression
- poor concentration, missing school, college or work
- lack of confidence, withdrawal from friends
- dependency or overinvolvement with parents, instead of developing independence.

It is important to remember that, if allowed to continue unchecked, both anorexia and bulimia can be life-threatening conditions. Over time, they are harder to treat, and the effects become more serious.

What is an eating disorder?

Worries about weight, shape and eating are common, especially among young girls. A lot of young people, many of whom are not overweight in the first place, want to be thinner. They often try to lose weight by dieting or skipping meals. For some, worries about weight become an obsession. This can turn into a serious eating disorder. This factsheet is about the most common eating disorders, anorexia nervosa and bulimia nervosa.

- Someone with anorexia nervosa worries all the time about being fat, even if they are skinny, and eats very little. They lose a lot of weight, and in girls their periods become irregular or stop.
- Someone with bulimia nervosa also worries a lot about weight. They alternate between eating next to nothing, and then having binges when they gorge themselves. They vomit or take laxatives to control their weight.

Both of these eating disorders are more common in girls, but do occur in boys. They can happen in young people of all backgrounds and cultures.

What causes eating disorders?

Eating disorders are caused by a number of different things.

- Worry or stress may lead to comfort eating. This may cause worries about getting fat.
- Dieting and missing meals leads to craving for food, loss of control and overeating.
- Anorexia or bulimia can develop as a complication of more extreme dieting, perhaps triggered by an upsetting event, such as family break-down, death or separation in the family, bullying at school or abuse.
- Sometimes, anorexia and bulimia may be a way of trying to feel in control if life feels stressful.
- More ordinary events such as the loss of a friend, a teasing remark or school exams may also be the trigger in a vulnerable person.

Who can develop an eating disorder?

Some of the factors which increase the likelihood of having an eating disorder include:

- being female
- being previously overweight
- lacking self-esteem
- being a perfectionist.

Young people with eating disorders often show obsessional behaviour.

Some people are more at risk than others. Sensitive or anxious individuals, who are having difficulty becoming independent from their families, are also more at risk. Eating disorders can also run in families. The families of young people with eating disorders often find change or conflict particularly difficult, and may be unusually close or overprotective.

Where can I get help?

If you think a young person may be developing an eating disorder, don't be afraid to ask them whether they are worried about themselves. Quite often young people with eating disorders are unable to acknowledge that there may be a problem, will not want you to interfere and may become angry or upset when you do. However, you may still be worried and you can seek advice from professionals in different agencies such as your GP or a paediatrician. It is important that you feel supported and not alone.

Janet, 18, writes

'Two years ago it was my "best friend" and now it's my "enemy"! It no longer controls me or my family and together we've pushed it away. I couldn't have done it alone. I wouldn't have made it to the unit if it wasn't for my mum and the school nurse who convinced me to see a professional team … that took them 6 months! … I was really pig-headed! I am talking about anorexia.

It started when I was 15 and my friends and I tried the "South Beach diet"… most of them dropped out but I stuck with it … I've always been competitive.

At home there was so much pressure to get "A" grades; at last, there was a different focus. I became obsessed with counting calories and even kept a food diary. I lost more weight but still felt huge and "ugly" and wanted to lose more … My friends tried to stop me and said they were worried, but I didn't care.

Slowly, I stopped going out with them, preferring to stay in and do my sit-up regime. I thought about taking slimming pills but was too scared so I bought laxatives instead. I felt so driven to lose weight; the thought of putting on an ounce scared me to death. I remember feeling weepy and very tired. At its worst, my fingers and toes went blue!

Then, I agreed to see the child and family mental health service where I met a team of professionals including a nurse, psychiatrist, psychologist and family therapist. They offered me individual therapy every week, to work through things and have my physical health monitored too. The family therapist was also able to offer us time as a family to work things out. This felt like the most important bit for a long time, especially for Dad who found it hard to understand anorexia. It was tough and sometimes we felt like throwing the towel in, but the team supported us and we felt safe. Even now some days are hard, but we got through it.' ✪

What can I do to help?

These simple suggestions are useful to help young people to maintain a healthy weight and avoid eating disorders.

- Ensure your child eats **regular meals**. The British Dietetic Association (www.bda.uk.com) recommends eating regularly throughout the day which usually means three main meals and three nutritious snacks in between such as fruit, yogurt or nuts. Too many sugary or high fat snacks should be avoided.

- Try to give a **'balanced' diet**, one that contains all the types of food your body needs, including carbohydrate foods such as bread, rice, pasta or cereals with every meal.

- **Don't let them miss meals** – long gaps encourage overeating.

- Encourage regular **exercise**.

- **Educate** your child not to be influenced by other people skipping meals or commenting on weight.

When is professional help needed?

When eating problems make family meals stressful, it is important to seek professional advice. Your GP will be able to advise you about what specialist help is available locally and arrange a referral. Help may be available through the paediatrician, dietitian or your local child and adolescent mental health service (CAMHS).

If the eating disorder causes physical ill health, it is essential to get medical help quickly. If untreated, there is a risk of infertility, thin bones (osteoporosis), stunted growth and even death, but if treated, most young people get better.

Annabelle's story

'I'm 16 now, but I think I started having a problem when I was 12. I became very worried about my weight and my body. I had put on a bit of weight and was very upset when a boy in my class called me fat. I remember feeling that even if I was doing very well in school, things weren't quite right and I wasn't quite good enough.

Gradually I ate less, lost masses of weight, but still believed that I was fat. Sometimes I "felt" fat and this made me feel very down. I stopped seeing most of my friends, and spent more and more time thinking about food and my body.

I was always checking the shape of my stomach and bottom – 20 or 30 times a day, looking at them in great detail. I felt very cold at times, and found it harder and harder to find the energy to do things as I was eating less and less.

I also weighed myself at least 5 times a day, and if my weight had not gone down, I checked my stomach, and tried dieting even more. Sometimes I binged on cakes and chocolate. I felt very guilty afterwards and would usually be sick so that I could get rid of the food and lose some weight. It felt as if I was going round and round in circles, with no means of escape.

One of my teachers noticed that I wasn't eating lunch and that I had become thin (or at least she thought I had). She spoke to my parents and I was taken to a clinic. At first I didn't want to know and I didn't want to be helped. However, I started a treatment called cognitive–behavioural therapy. I learned to look at the links between my thoughts, feelings and behaviour, but more importantly, I learned that I could eat regularly, without putting on weight.

Gradually, I put on some weight and worked on my checking and weighing behaviour. It wasn't easy to get better. I slowly started to eat the foods that I used to avoid. Sometimes I still find myself thinking the way I used to, but now I know that this is only one way of thinking, one way of being, and most of the time choose not to do this.

I love going out clubbing with my friends now and I don't argue quite so much with my parents, well at least not about food anyway.' ✪

Recommended reading

Other factsheets in this series:
The emotional cost of bullying,
CBT (for young people), Worries
and anxieties, CAMHS

*Anorexia Nervosa: A Guide for
Sufferers and Their Families*,
by R. L. Palmer. Published by
Penguin Books, 1989.

*Anorexia Nervosa: A Survival
Guide For Families, Friends And
Sufferers*, by Janet Treasure.
Published by Psychology Press,
1997.

National Institute for Health and
Clinical Excellence. *Eating
Disorders: Information for the
Public* (CG9). 2004.

*The Young Mind: An Essential
Guide to Mental Health for
Young Adults, Parents and
Teachers*, edited by Sue Bailey
and Mike Shooter (2009) –
an accessible, user-friendly
handbook produced by the
Royal College of Psychiatrists.

References

National Institute for Health and
Clinical Excellence. *Eating
Disorders: Core Interventions in
the Treatment and Management
of Anorexia Nervosa, Bulimia
Nervosa and Related Eating
Disorders*. NICE, 2004.

Rutter M, Bishop D, Pine D, et al (eds)
*Rutter's Child and Adolescent
Psychiatry* (5th edn). Wiley–
Blackwell, 2008.

Useful websites

➲ **B-eat (beating eating disorders)**: www.b-eat.co.uk;
helpline for parents: 0845 634 1414.

➲ **YoungMinds**: www.youngminds.org.uk; for any adult
concerned about the emotions and behaviour of a child or
young person. Parents' helpline: 0808 802 5544. .

➲ **King's College London**: www.kcl.ac.uk/iop/depts/pm/
research/eatingdisorders/index.aspx; website with up-to-date
information on eating disorders and various other disorders.

Notes

For a catalogue of public education materials or copies of our leaflets contact: Book Sales/Leaflets, The Royal College of Psychiatrists, 17 Belgrave Square, London SW1X 8PG. Email: leaflets@rcpsych.ac.uk, tel: 020 7235 2351 ext. 6146.

Revised by the Royal College of Psychiatrists' Child and Family Public Education Editorial Board. With grateful thanks to Dr Vasu Balaguru. This leaflet reflects the best possible evidence at the time of writing.

26 Chronic physical illness: the effects on mental health

Information for parents, carers and anyone who works with young people

This is one in a series of factsheets for parents, teachers and anyone who works with young people, with practical, up-to-date information about mental health problems (emotional, behavioural and psychiatric disorders) that can affect children and young people.

This factsheet looks at the effects that a long physical illness can have on a young person's mental health, and offers advice about how to recognise and deal with these problems.

Why are mental health problems so common?

Serious illness or disability can cause a lot of work and stress for everyone in the family, especially the parents. Children who are ill have many more stressful experiences than children without an illness. Most children will, at some time, get upset by this. Sometimes, the upset feelings and behaviour can go on and on. If they do, this can add to the child's health problems by making their life even more difficult.

How does this affect the child and family?

Following the diagnosis of a potentially serious or long-term illness, most parents and children will go through a process of coming to terms with it.

> **How does physical illness affect a child's mental health?**
>
> Children with a long-lasting physical illness are at least twice as likely to experience emotional problems or disturbed behaviour. This is especially true of physical illnesses that involve the brain, such as epilepsy and cerebral palsy.

Long-term effects

- The affected child might have **fewer opportunities** to learn everyday skills and to develop their interests and hobbies.
- **Problems at school** are also common. Be sure to be in touch with your child's teacher on a regular basis.
    - Your child might have to miss a lot of school and have particular difficulties with learning. They might need extra help at school.
    - Your child might see themselves as different from other children, and they may hate this.
    - Some children may become depressed.
    - Some children may be vulnerable to bullying.
- It is easy for you as parents to be **overprotective** of your child. You may find it harder to say 'no' than you normally would, making it difficult to control your child. It is harder to allow them to manage the rough-and-tumble of childhood.
- Sometimes it can be difficult and **confusing** to cope with all the different doctors and other professionals involved with your child's illness. This can be very stressful for everyone.
- **Brothers and sisters** sometimes feel that they are being neglected. They may feel embarrassed by their ill brother or sister. They may also feel responsible for them. They can miss out on school or their social life, get bullied or lose friendships. Therefore, it is important to consider how all members of the family are challenged and affected when a child has a long-lasting illness.

What can I do to help?

It is very important to remember that although long-lasting illness does make things very difficult, most children and their families cope well. It is only a minority who experience problems.

- Live as normal a life as possible.
- Be open with your child about their difficulties.
- Restrict them as little as possible.

- Help them to get out and about with other children of their own age.
- Encourage your child to be as independent as possible.
- Meet other families with similar experiences.
- Seek help if you feel that you are not managing.

A lot can be done to prevent further problems developing. Parents who understand the emotional impact of the illness on the child and on the rest of the family are much better placed to spot problems early, and do something about them.

Where can I get help?

Making sure that there is enough help and support is very important. In addition to support from family and friends, try:

- Contact a Family (see 'Useful websites' for contact details)
- you child's paediatrician
- your GP
- voluntary support groups
- Social Services
- school
- health visitor
- school nurse.

If there are signs that your child is developing emotional or behavioural problems, speak to your child's GP/paediatrician/specialist. They can advise you or refer your child to the mental health liaison team in the hospital or to the child and adolescent mental health service (CAMHS) who will have experience in managing young people with both physical and emotional/behavioural difficulties.

Child mental health professionals can help with the emotional and psychological aspects of the illness. Following assessment, they may offer family work and/or individual talking therapy for your child. They will also want to work jointly with other professionals involved in the child's care, and with staff from the young person's school. This can help sort out any problems related to the treatment, and make sure that everyone is working together effectively.

Sean, 12, talks about his diabetes

'When the doctor told my mum I had diabetes, I couldn't understand why she got so upset. It wasn't going to kill me or anything – not like a girl in our school who had cancer…then I didn't understand how much I'd have to take care of what I ate…or at least I'd have to work out how much insulin I had to take…I couldn't just relax.

Then there were the injections and the "pen" for testing my blood sugar. They don't exactly hurt, but it's a bit like being a prisoner…having to do it all the time. Then sometimes I get fed up and think, "Why should I have to do it and why did it happen to me anyway?" The doctors say it wasn't anything I did or even my mum or dad did, but I can't often believe this, it must have been someone's fault…and if I do play about with it a bit…I know it really winds my mum up…I know I sometimes do it on purpose when she'd been winding me up. Dad just gets angry when I do it, and sometimes it leads to arguments…I mean arguments between them. But then they sort of get together and gang up on me. Sometimes I even thought I could get them to stop arguing by playing around with my BMs [blood sugar measurements], and a few times it worked. Funny really…I felt like a winner…I mean that I was in charge when that happened.

The hospital told me I might have problems if I didn't try to get better control of my BMs, and one doctor wanted to take me up to the adult ward to see the people who'd lost toes or couldn't see properly. No way, I said. Still, I did later talk to the diabetes nurse and a nurse from the mental health team. They were really great, but after I talked to them I sort of lost the fun out of mucking about with the BMs. I realised that I would be better off taking better care of my diabetes and felt a bit more relaxed about the injections.' ✪

Recommended reading

Other factsheets in this series:
Depression (for young people),
The emotional cost of bullying,
CAMHS

References

Glazebrook C, Hollis C, Heussler
    H, et al. Detecting emotional
    and behavioural problems in
    paediatric clinics. *Child Care
    Health Dev* 2003; 29: 141–9.

Hysing M, Elgen I, Gillberg G,
    et al. Chronic physical illness
    and mental health in children.
    Results from a large-scale
    population study. *J Child
    Psychol Psychiatry Allied Disc*
    2007; 48: 785–92.

Rutter M, Bishop D, Pine D, et al (eds)
    *Rutter's Child and Adolescent
    Psychiatry* (5th edn). Wiley–
    Blackwell, 2008.

Useful websites

- **Contact a Family**: www.cafamily.org.uk; support for families with children with a disability. Helpline: 0808 808 3555.

- **The Back-Up Trust**: www.backuptrust.org.uk; a national charity supporting people paralysed through spinal cord injury.

- **YoungMinds**: www.youngminds.org.uk; information and advice on child mental health issue and a parents' helpline: 0808 802 5544

Notes

....

....

....

....

....

....

....

....

....

Medically unexplained physical symptoms

Information for parents, carers and anyone who works with young people

This is one in a series of factsheets for parents, teachers and anyone who works with young people, with practical, up-to-date information about mental health problems (emotional, behavioural and psychiatric disorders) that can affect children and young people.

This factsheet looks at why some young people have problematic physical symptoms when there seems to be no physical cause. It also offers advice about how to recognise and manage these problems.

What are the causes?

Physical illness or injury may be a factor at the beginning, but when no obvious physical explanation can be found, emotional or psychological factors need to be thought about.

These problems are more common in children and young people who:

- are feeling stressed, for instance about moving school, friendship problems or not managing schoolwork
- are very sensitive to physical symptoms and pain
- are very sensitive to others
- have low self-esteem
- tend to be fussy or perfectionist
- are very anxious and worry more than most
- worry continuously about the symptoms and their effects on everyday activities – this can cause the symptoms to continue, and even get worse.

Unexplained physical symptoms may also be part of another psychiatric condition, such as depression or anxiety. There may also be a family history of unexplained physical symptoms.

What are the effects of unexplained physical symptoms?

For most children and young people, with appropriate reassurance, the symptoms are short lived. However, for some, everyday life can become very uncomfortable and stressful. Unexplained physical symptoms can also be very worrying for parents.

The symptoms may result in young people:

- missing a lot of school; they may not achieve what they should socially and academically
- seeing less of their friends – this means fewer interests, hobbies and fun
- becoming anxious and depressed
- being less independent than other young people their age.

Who can help?

- Your **GP** will be able to assess your child and help decide whether any specialist investigation or treatment is required. If necessary, they will refer your child to the local paediatrician or child and adolescent mental health service (CAMHS).
- **Specialists**, such as psychiatrists, can help identify the psychological factors that may be contributing to the symptoms, and can also help to distinguish unexplained physical symptoms from other mental health problems, such as depression.
- **Talking treatments** can help you and your child to manage unexplained physical symptoms better.
- **Medication** can also play a part, particularly in treating any anxiety and depression that the child may also be experiencing.

What are medically unexplained symptoms?

Medically unexplained physical symptoms (MUPS) are when someone suffers from physical symptoms for which no underlying physical cause can be found.

About one in ten children and adolescents have this condition. Common symptoms are headaches, stomach aches, joint pains and tiredness. Less commonly, young people can have significant unexplained physical symptoms, including muscle weakness, collapses, 'fit-like' episodes, and severe and chronic pain.

How is it treated?

A **planned approach** to treat the symptoms is important. The aim of the treatment is to help your child to recover gradually by creating more effective ways of coping with the symptoms, and getting back to a normal daily routine.

Everyone needs to **work together** as a team towards the same goals: you, your child, the paediatrician, psychiatrist, GP and school may all need to get involved.

It can be helpful for everyone involved in helping the child to meet and **review their progress** from time to time. This allows ideas to be shared about the best ways forward – physical, psychological and educational.

For the most severe unexplained physical symptoms, **specialist help** through CAMHS may be needed to develop a planned approach to the problem.

Caring for a young person with unexplained physical symptoms can be very stressful. Family life can become dominated by your child's difficulties. Parents will need to be **caring**, but also **determined** and **positive**, even when things seem bleak and uncertain.

Often parents find it hard to know what to do for the best – when to encourage and when to comfort, when to insist and when to take the pressure off. You may benefit from expert help and advice about this.

Treatment is best done with active participation from the whole family. It will involve:

- finding ways of paying less attention to the symptoms
- a small, but steady, increase in everyday and social activities for the child/young person
- the young person will be encouraged to do more for themselves and to regain their confidence and independence
- asking teachers to help with looking at ways of overcoming any school or education problems.

Family or individual counselling may be helpful if it is focused on issues such as how to:

- respond to pain and other symptoms more effectively
- increase levels of physical and social activity
- manage depression, anxiety, lack of confidence and poor motivation
- deal with family relationship difficulties when these become part of the problem.

Callum, 17, talks about his unexplained seizures

'It all started when I was in year 9. I'd always had difficulties getting on with the other boys at my all-boys independent school. I didn't really fit in with the whole rugby thing, which was the main focus for many of the boys. This became an increasing problem. I was teased and intimidated in the changing rooms before PE and games. I then started to develop really bad headaches and my GP gave me painkillers. The headaches got worse and I started to get double vision. Mum and Dad got really worried about me. I kept going to the GP who said there was nothing wrong with me. I felt I was wasting his time.

Things got worse at school and just before my end-of-year exams. I had a fit at school and I was taken to our local hospital where they did loads of tests but couldn't find anything wrong. I stayed in hospital for a week but when I went home the fits started again. My paediatrician said the fits weren't caused by epilepsy and he suggested we invite someone from CAMHS [child and adolescent mental health service] to come to my appointment. I was not sure about this but my parents thought it would be worth a try.

I then met one of CAMHS' psychologists who wasn't what I was expecting at all. He was really helpful. He helped me and my family make sense of my fits. It took a while for the fits to stop and we had to put lots of plans in to support me at school, but in the end they went away. I'm now attending sixth form at a different school and I am hoping to get a place at university.' ✪

Recommended reading

Other factsheets in this series: Worries and anxieties, The emotional cost of bullying, Eating disorders, CAMHS

The Young Mind: An Essential Guide to Mental Health for Young Adults, Parents and Teachers, edited by Sue Bailey and Mike Shooter (2009) – an accessible, user-friendly handbook produced by the Royal College of Psychiatrists.

References

Eminson DM. Somatising in children and adolescents. 1: Clinical presentations and aetiological factors. *Adv Psychiatr Treat* 2001; 7: 266–74.

Eminson DM. Somatising in children and adolescents. 2: Management and outcomes. *Adv Psychiatr Treat* 2001; 7: 388–98.

Garralda ME. Practitioner review. Assessment and management of somatisation in childhood and adolescence: a practical perspective. *J Child Psychol Psychiatry Allied Disc* 1999; 40: 1159–67.

Garralda ME. The links between somatisation in children and adults. In *Family Matters: Interfaces Between Child and Adult Mental Health* (eds P Reder, M McClure, A Jolley): 122–231. Routledge, 2000.

Taylor S, Garralda E. The management of somatoform disorder in childhood. *Curr Opin Psychiatry* 2003; 16: 227–31.

Useful websites

- **ChildLine**: www.childline.org.uk; provides a free and confidential telephone service for children. Helpline: 0800 1111.
- **Mental Health Foundation**: www.mentalhealth.org.uk; charity involved in improving the lives of people with mental health problems or intellectual disabilities.
- **Young Minds**: www.youngminds.org.uk; provides information and advice on child mental health issues. Parents' helpline: 0808 802 5544.

Notes

28 Chronic fatigue syndrome: helping your child get better

Information for parents, carers and anyone who works with young people

This is one in a series of factsheets for parents, teachers and anyone who works with young people, with practical, up-to-date information about mental health problems (emotional, behavioural and psychiatric disorders) that can affect children and young people.

This factsheet aims to explain what chronic fatigue syndrome is, its causes and symptoms, and offers practical advice about how to get help for a young person who is affected by it.

What are the symptoms?

The main symptom is extreme tiredness (fatigue) after little effort, which is not improved by rest, and not explained by physical or psychiatric illness. Chronic fatigue syndrome commonly starts with a short or sudden illness such as 'flu' or glandular fever, but it can also start gradually. It is a severely disabling condition that can often last a long time or comes and goes.

Common symptoms include:

- headaches
- aching muscles and other bodily pains
- disruption of your child's usual sleeping and eating patterns.

Like other severe physical illnesses, chronic fatigue syndrome has some important emotional and psychological effects. The child may become depressed, irritable and anxious, and find it difficult to concentrate or remember things.

Chronic fatigue syndrome can be a difficult diagnosis to make. Children often receive repeated specialist medical investigations.

> ### What is chronic fatigue syndrome?
> Chronic fatigue syndrome is a rare condition that usually starts in the mid-teens but can occur earlier (rarely before the age of 7). It has also been called myalgic encephalomyelitis (ME).

What are the effects of chronic fatigue syndrome?

The disorder can seriously disrupt normal life. Your child may be unable to:

- carry out their usual activities, including attending school
- go out and see friends
- carry on with their hobbies.

School can be very difficult to cope with. Young people with chronic fatigue syndrome may quickly become very unfit from staying in bed, or just doing not very much for a long time. This causes rapid muscle loss, even in healthy people. All these complications make recovery more difficult.

Everyone in the family can feel the strain. Sometimes a parent may have to give up work to nurse their sick child. Brothers and sisters may feel that they are being neglected. Parents may disagree about whether the child is really sick, or is just 'attention-seeking'.

How can I get help?

In the early stages of the illness, it may seem that no one knows what the problem is and how to solve it. This can upset the child, who may feel that no one believes that they are ill or understands them. Relationships can become strained at home and at school.

Your GP or school doctor will be able to refer your child to a paediatrician or child psychiatrist working in your local child and adolescent mental health service (CAMHS) for assessment and treatment. The school, especially the school nurse and psychologist, may need to support your child with problems at school.

Jess, 14

'It started when I was off school with a bad sore throat. I felt so tired. I found it difficult to get out of bed in the morning and slept in the afternoon but then slept for hours at night.

I used to be really good at tennis and I was in nearly all the top sets at school. I really wanted to get back to school because I knew I was getting behind. My friends came round to see me after I was ill, but I felt so tired that I could only see them for a short time, so they have now stopped ringing and coming round. I do miss them but I feel too tired to contact them. If I do anything, I need time to rest. The other day I went out to the shops with Mum and Dad but then it took me 3 days to recover.

Over the past few years I have had many different tests but nothing has been found. It has helped talking to my school about starting to do some work at home. My mum and I were very worried about doing any exercises, but the physiotherapist has visited me at home and she understands my fear of getting worse. So I have agreed that she will help me with some gentle exercises.

My doctor suggested seeing a psychiatrist but I didn't think I had a mental illness. However, my GP explained to me and I began to realise that I have been ill for so long that perhaps it might help me and my family to talk to a therapist about this. I agreed to see a therapist at CAMHS to see what they could do. We have been seeing a family therapist at CAMHS and I feel it is helping all of us to talk about our difficulties and feel more positive about each other.' ✪

How is chronic fatigue syndrome treated?

The overall aim is to help the child or young person with chronic fatigue syndrome to gradually resume normal activities. There has been some controversy about how best to treat children with chronic fatigue syndrome.

- **Combined therapy**

  Research looking at various approaches to treatment suggests a combination of approaches including cognitive–behavioural therapy (CBT) and graded exercise therapy, and does not specifically support any one type of treatment. A programme of gradually increasing gentle activity can help to rebuild your child's muscles and fitness.

- **Family and school engagement**

  Family or individual talking therapy can help in overcoming depression, anxiety, lack of confidence, poor motivation, or family and relationship problems. It is also important to look at ways of getting your child to continue their education by speaking to the school/teachers.

- **Support**

  Although it can be hard to know when and how to encourage your child and when to comfort them, it is important to try to maintain a supportive and positive outlook.

- **Specialist involvement**

  You may find expert advice from your child's paediatrician, child psychiatrist, CAMHS team and education staff helpful. It is also a good idea for everyone involved in helping your child with chronic fatigue syndrome to meet together to talk about progress from time to time. This allows everyone to share ideas about the best ways forward: physical, psychological and educational. Working as a team is important and a regular review of progress is essential.

  Research looking at how children recover has shown that the majority of severely affected children make a complete recovery, and others improve sufficiently to lead near normal lives.

Useful websites

⊃ **Young Minds**: www.youngminds.org.uk; provides information and advice on child mental health issues. Parents' helpline: 0808 802 5544.

⊃ **AYME** (pronounced 'aim'): www.ayme.org.uk; a national charity for children and young people with chronic fatigue syndrome aged 5–25.

⊃ **Tymes Trust: The Young ME Sufferers Trust**: www.tymestrust.org; national UK service for children and young people with ME (chronic fatigue syndrome) and their families.

Recommended reading

Other factsheets in this series:
Chronic physical illness, Medically unexplained physical symptoms, CBT (for young people), CAMHS

Self Help for Chronic Fatigue Syndrome: A Guide for Young People, by T. Chalder & K. Hussain. Blue Stallion Publications, 2002.

The Young Mind: An Essential Guide to Mental Health for Young Adults, Parents and Teachers, edited by Sue Bailey and Mike Shooter (2009) – an accessible, user-friendly handbook produced by the Royal College of Psychiatrists.

References

National Institute for Health and Clinical Excellence. *Chronic Fatigue Syndrome/Myalgic Encephalomyelitis (or Encephalopathy); Diagnosis and Management* (CG53). NICE, 2007.

Rangel L, Garralda ME, Levin M, et al. The course of severe chronic fatigue syndrome in childhood. *J Royal Soc Med* 2000; 93: 129–34.

Royal College of Paediatrics and Child Health. *Evidence Based Guideline for the Management of CFS/ME (Chronic Fatigue Syndrome/Myalgic Encephalopathy) in Children and Young People* (2008 update). RCPCH, 2008.

Rutter M, Bishop D, Pine D, et al (eds) *Rutter's Child and Adolescent Psychiatry* (5th edn). Wiley–Blackwell, 2008.

Viner R, Gregorowski A, Wine C, et al. Outpatient rehabilitative treatment of chronic fatigue syndrome (CFS/ME). *Arch Dis Child* 2004; 89: 615–9.

Whiting P, Bagnall AM, Sowden AJ, et al. Interventions for the treatment and management of chronic fatigue syndrome: a systematic review. *JAMA* 2001; 286: 1360–8.

Notes

29 Parental mental illness: the problems for children
Information for parents, carers and anyone who works with young people

This is one in a series of factsheets for parents, teachers and anyone who works with young people, with practical, up-to-date information about mental health problems (emotional, behavioural and psychiatric disorders) that can affect children and young people.

This factsheet provides information on the difficulties faced by children who have a parent with a mental illness, and gives some practical advice as to how to deal with those.

How many children have a parent with mental illness?

Many children will grow up with a parent who, at some point, will have some degree of mental illness. Most of these parents will have mild or short-lived illnesses, and will usually be treated by their GP.

A few children live with a parent who has a severe mental illness such as schizophrenia or bipolar disorder. In fact, 68% of women and 57% of men with a mental illness are parents. In addition, many children live with a parent who has long-term mental health problems, as well as alcohol or drug problems and personality disorders.

Why do children living with a parent with mental illness have difficulties?

Children can often cope well with all sorts of life upsets, especially if:

- the problem is short lived and does not keep repeating
- they can understand what is happening and, as much as possible, understand why it is happening.

Parents cannot control the fact that some illnesses, especially mental illnesses, can last a long time and may come back. Some parents may try to protect their children from their illness by keeping it a secret or treating it as something which cannot be asked about or explained. Although this is often done for good reasons, it is a mistake and can make it more difficult for the children to cope with or manage their own feelings. Such a situation may create a number of problems for children.

- They may worry that they are to blame for their parent's illness and they may feel depressed.
- They may develop the same illness. Although for some conditions the risk of having a similar illness can be higher within families, this can be reduced if the child is helped to see that they are not part of the illness, and they are able to have a good relationship with their parents, peers or any other adults who can be trusted and help them. Understanding the illness helps the child to achieve this.

What is mental illness?

Mental illness is an illness of the mind in which a person to some degree loses control over aspects of their thoughts and/or their feelings. It can be very mild, such as mild depression when things look much worse than they are, or very severe, for example when a person's life is totally dominated by an illness such as schizophrenia and they cannot live independently.

It is estimated that mental illness will affect one in four of us at some time in our lives. When a person is mentally healthy they feel good about themselves; they can do everyday things easily, such as going to school or work and enjoying their hobbies and friends. Even when things go wrong, they can usually sort it out themselves, although this may not be easy.

When someone has a mental illness, they may find everyday things very difficult to do and they may feel confused and upset a lot of the time. They may do things that seem normal to them, but to other people watching they may seem strange.

For some children it may be more difficult to cope when they:

- are separated again and again from a parent who needs to go into hospital for treatment
- are living with a parent who is very unwell and treated at home
- feel unsure of their relationship with the parent with a mental illness
- are not being looked after properly
- are being hit or mistreated (this is more likely if the parent has alcohol or drug problems or personality difficulties)
- are having to look after an ill parent, or are taking care of brothers and sisters, and missing school

- are being teased or bullied by others
- hear unkind things being said about their ill parent.

Even when children have all the right support and explanation, they may still at times feel upset, frightened, worried by or ashamed of their parent's illness or behaviour.

What problems can children develop?

Some children withdraw into themselves, become anxious and find it hard to concentrate on their schoolwork. They may find it very difficult to talk about their parent's illness or their problems, especially when they have had no explanation of their illness. This may stop them from getting help. Children are often ashamed of their parent's illness and worry about becoming ill themselves. They can be preoccupied with fears of 'catching' the illness and some children can show signs of a similar illness or severe emotional problems.

Children can have physical health problems and struggle with school and their education, especially when they live with parents in poverty, poor housing or have an unstable life.

What can I do to help?

There are some steps that can be taken to help avoid these problems and to make the child or young person's life easier. For example:

- having a reliable, consistent and caring parent or other adult they can talk to
- being given information and an explanation about their parent's illness
- encouraging and supporting the child in their everyday routine, such as attending school, playing and doing things like their peers do.

If you are a parent with a mental health problem, it is important that you make sure you have the right help. You can discuss your child's needs for care and support, especially when you are unwell, with your doctor or the professional treating you. All mental health professionals involved in the care of an ill parent should ask about the needs of the children in the household, and whether any further help is required, even if the parent is not being treated in hospital.

A child may really value the chance to talk about their parent's illness and their own fears with a professional who is familiar with these things.

It is important for parents and teachers to be aware of the possible stresses on the young person with an ill parent, and to recognise that a child's difficult behaviour may be a cry for help.

- The GP or a social worker can organise support and practical help for the family in caring for the child or young person, and give advice and work with other professionals if there are problems that are harming the child's health or development.

Susie, 11

Susie is 11 and her school attendance is irregular. When in school, she is often tired, dressed untidily and her hair looks dirty. She is quite a 'bossy' girl and has difficulty making friends. Some of the younger children feel bullied and intimidated by her, and the school is getting more and more worried about her behaviour.

Susie's mum is a single parent and has twice been invited to come to school to discuss Susie's behaviour and attendance, but she has not turned up on either occasion. An educational welfare officer is allocated to the case. On a home visit the officer finds out that the mum has bipolar disorder. She has medication but does not always take it, which results in good and bad days, and accounts for Susie's erratic attendance.

The reason for Susie's bossy behaviour also soon becomes apparent as she needs to 'boss' her mum to get her to take her medication. As well as looking after her mum's well-being, she is trying to be a parent to her 9-year-old brother, Will.

The local community mental health team reviews Susie's mum's case and assess both the management of her illness and her needs as a parent. The team sets up a monitoring process to ensure she takes her medication. Susie's mum agrees to start attending a voluntary drop-in day centre, once a week, to seek support and advice on self-managing her condition. Both children are assessed under the common assessment framework and support is offered to them.

The behaviour support team meets with the school to implement a plan to support Susie to reduce her bossy behaviour and monitor her attendance. She is also given learning support to help to catch up with work she has missed. The educational welfare officer also contacts the local young carers' project to see whether Susie can get support from them. It is decided that the services she needs are befriending and attending the homework club. The project will also give her information about bipolar disorder. Will is offered a place at the local church Saturday activity club and is also given information about bipolar disorder. ✪

- The child could join a local group (sometimes also called 'young carers') specifically for the children and young people who care for their parents or siblings.

- Some children may be offered therapy or counselling. A lot of children will not be very happy about this as they assume it means that they are either the 'problem' or that they will develop the illness. Young carers' groups avoid this problem as the children are respected as helping their parent.

- If the child or young person has severe emotional or behavioural problems that interfere with their life and that don't seem to be improving, more specialist help may be needed. Their GP will be able to advise about local services and to refer a young person, if necessary, to the local child and adolescent mental health service (CAMHS). This service usually includes child and adolescent psychiatrists, psychologists, psychotherapists, nurses and social workers.

Recommended reading

Other factsheets in this series: Worries and anxieties, CAMHS

Minds, Myths and ME booklet, produced by four British young carers, available from the Royal College of Psychiatrists: www.rcpsych.ac.uk/mentalhealthinfo/youngpeople/caringforyoungcarers.aspx

The Young Mind: An Essential Guide to Mental Health for Young Adults, Parents and Teachers, edited by Sue Bailey and Mike Shooter (2009) – an accessible, user-friendly handbook produced by the Royal College of Psychiatrists.

'When a parent has a mental illness', a film for young carers by Dr Aland Cooklin, also available from the Royal College of Psychiatrists: www.rcpsych.ac.uk/mentalhealthinfoforall/youngpeople/caringforaparent.aspx

References

Cooklin A. *Being Seen and Heard: The Needs of Children of Parents With Mental Illness* (DVD & CD). RCPsych Publications, 2006.

Gopfert M, Webster J, Seeman M (eds) *Parental Psychiatric Disorder: Distressed Parents and Their Families* (2nd edn). Cambridge University Press, 2004.

Useful websites

⊃ **Bipolar UK**: www.bipolaruk.org.uk; supports people with a diagnosis of bipolar disorder and their families.

⊃ **Carers Trust**: www.carers.org; information and support about being a carer and a young carer, including information about local groups. There is also a website for young carers: www.youngcarers.net

⊃ **Rethink Mental Illness**: www.rethink.org; information and advice to people with severe mental illness and their carers.

Notes

....

....

....

....

....

....

....

30 Who's who in CAMHS
Information for parents, carers and anyone who works with young people

This is one in a series of factsheets for parents, teachers and anyone who works with young people, with practical, up-to-date information about mental health problems (emotional, behavioural and psychiatric disorders) that can affect children and young people.

This factsheet describes who works in child and adolescent mental health services (CAMHS), what they do and how they may be able to help if you or someone you know has a mental health problem.

Where can I find CAMHS?

Services in CAMHS are organised into four tiers. Many people when they talk about CAMHS mean tier 3 services – the community CAMHS teams. But CAMHS professionals can work in one or more of the following places:

- community CAMHS clinics (also called tier 3 services)
- out-patient clinics or alongside paediatricians in general hospitals
- specialised in-patient, day patient or out-patient units (tier 4 services)
- in schools and some GP practices (tier 2 services)
- alongside Social Services or youth offending services (YOS)
- in children's centres.

In addition to offering appointments in the above places, some CAMHS professionals can see you at home if it is difficult for you to meet elsewhere.

> **What is CAMHS?**
>
> Child and adolescent mental health services, in short called CAMHS, come in all shapes and sizes. They are made up of different mental health professionals, all working together to help young people and their families where there are mental health problems.

Who works in CAMHS?

The different child mental health professionals in the team usually include:

- **child and adolescent psychiatrists** – they are medically qualified doctors who specialise in working with young people with mental health problems and their families
- **clinical psychologists** – they can assess and help with children's psychological functioning, emotional well-being and development
- **child psychotherapists** – they are trained therapists who work with children helping to deal with their emotional and mental health problems
- **family therapists** – they are trained therapists who work with children and their families together to help them understand and manage the difficulties that are happening in their lives
- **social workers** – they are trained to help children and families who need extra support or help to keep them safe
- **mental health practitioners** – they are usually trained in mental health and help in the assessment (understanding) and management of emotional, behavioural and mental health problems.

Some teams can have other professionals such as paediatricians, educational psychologists, art therapists, and speech and language therapists.

All CAMHS professionals are trained and experienced in working with young people with mental health problems. They may also have some specialist skills, which they may use for specific conditions or treatments.

What problems can they help with?

Many children and young people are troubled by emotional, behavioural and psychiatric problems. These can cause worry and distress both to themselves and to those who care for them.

Professionals working in CAMHS deal with a wide range of mental health problems including all those addressed in these factsheets and many more.

A large part of CAMHS professionals' work is to:

- identify the problem
- understand the causes
- advise about what may help.

Child psychiatrists are the only CAMHS professionals who can prescribe medication if it is needed. Sometimes, specially trained CAMHS nurses may prescribe for some illnesses (e.g. attention-deficit hyperactivity disorder (ADHD)). Other CAMHS professionals, for example child psychotherapists, psychologists and family therapists, are particularly skilled in providing talking therapies of different sorts. Most of the work that they do with children, young people and their families is done through out-patient appointments, while the young person continues to live at home.

Child and adolescent mental health professionals are sometimes asked to provide expert opinion to the courts about child welfare issues.

How can I be seen in CAMHS?

Your GP, health visitor, paediatrician, school doctor or nurse, educational psychologist, special educational needs coordinating officer (SENCO) in school, or social worker will be able to discuss any concerns and arrange for an appointment in a CAMHS clinic, if necessary.

Recommended reading

CAMHS Inside Out: A Young Person's Guide to Child and Adolescent Mental Health Services. A booklet and a leaflet to tell young people more about what to expect from CAMHS; it can be downloaded from www.rcpsych. ac.uk/quality/qualityandaccreditation/qinmaccamhs/youngperson-sguidetocamhs.aspx

Reference

Department of Health. *Standard 9: The Mental Health and Psychological Well-Being of Children and Young People*. Department of Health, 2004.

Useful website

⊃ **Young Minds**: www.youngminds.org.uk; free advice and support for parents worried about their children's behaviour, emotional problems and mental health. Parents' Helpline: 0808 802 5544.

Notes

....

....

....

....

....

Liv, 15, talks about her experience of CAMHS

'I suppose I wasn't really me for quite a while before people noticed. In the end it was school; Mum and Dad were always far too busy to see what was really happening. I was being really short with everyone, teachers, even my friends; I fell out with quite a few people. I was picking fights, but I didn't know why. It was almost like it gave me an excuse to be able to shout and scream at someone.

My English teacher asked me to pop in to see our school nurse. After seeing me a few times, the nurse said she was worried about me and wanted me to see someone. She mentioned CAMHS. I didn't know what that meant; when she explained, I got quite cross. I told her I wasn't mad, I didn't need a shrink.

I went though, just to see if they would be any use. I met a doctor, a psychiatrist, first. But it wasn't like seeing any doctors I'd met before. We sat in chairs and had a really long talk. That was all. Then I went again and the same thing happened. Over a few weeks I managed to tell the doctor about what was going on at home; Mum and Dad, the arguing. She wondered about asking the whole family to come to a meeting.

They all came. The doctor was there, but she asked someone she works with, a family therapist, to join us too. They got my little sister to talk, which was amazing because she said she wouldn't say a thing. They got everyone to say something, somehow, without them really noticing. Mum was in tears when my sister said she didn't like seeing her so sad all the time. I was so relieved. They would really see now that it wasn't just me. It was all of us.' ✪

For a catalogue of public education materials or copies of our leaflets contact: Book Sales/Leaflets, The Royal College of Psychiatrists, 17 Belgrave Square, London SW1X 8PG. Email: leaflets@rcpsych.ac.uk, tel: 020 7235 2351 ext. 6146.

Revised by the Royal College of Psychiatrists' Child and Family Public Education Editorial Board. This leaflet reflects the best possible evidence at the time of writing. The Royal College of Psychiatrists is a charity registered in England and Wales (228636) and in Scotland (SC038369). © The Royal College of Psychiatrists 2013

31 Surviving adolescence
A toolkit for parents, teachers, young people and anyone who works with young people

This toolkit is mainly for the parents and carers of teenagers, but we hope that teenagers might also enjoy reading it. It gives information about what happens to a young person in adolescence, the upheavals it can cause, some of the problems that arise, and ways in which they can be managed.

What changes occur in adolescence?

Rapid changes can occur physically and emotionally. There are also changes socially (attending secondary school, spending more time with peers) which can present with new challenges such as using drugs/alcohol and sexual relationships.

Physical: hormones, timing and changes

The process of rapid physical changes in adolescence is called **puberty**. It starts gradually, from around 11 years for girls and 13 years for boys. The age at which puberty starts has been dropping in most countries, probably owing to better nutrition. So, your children may hit puberty earlier than you did.

The **hormone changes** responsible actually begin some years earlier and may produce periods of moodiness and restlessness. Girls start these changes before boys and will, for the first 3 or 4 years, appear to be maturing much faster. After this, boys catch up.

These changes are:

- in girls: menstrual periods, growth of under-arm, body and pubic hair
- in boys: voice breaks (becomes deeper), growth of body, pubic and facial hair, erections and wet dreams
- in both: rapid physical growth.

By the age of 17, they will be young men and women who may be bigger than their parents and capable of having children themselves. In spite of this, they often still need **support from you**.

It is not surprising that, with the speed of these changes, some adolescents become very concerned about their appearance. They may feel worried, especially if these changes happen earlier or later than in their peers. It is important to remember that there is a lot of difference in the ages at which these changes happen, and adolescents need to be reassured about this.

Growth and development uses a lot of energy, and this may be why teenagers often seem to need so much sleep. Their getting up late may be irritating, but it may well not be just laziness.

Psychological and emotional changes

As well as growing taller, starting to shave or having periods, people of this age start to **think and feel differently**. They make close relationships outside the family, with friends of their own age. Relationships within the family also change. Parents become less important in their children's eyes, as their life outside the family develops.

Real **disagreements** emerge for the first time as young people develop views of their own that may not be shared by their parents. Adolescents spend a lot of time in each other's company, or on the telephone or internet chatting to each other. Although this can be irritating to parents, it is an important way of becoming more **independent**. These friendships are part of learning how to get on with other people, and gaining a sense of **identity** that is distinct from that of the family. Clothes and **appearance** are a way of expressing solidarity with friends, although teenage children are still more likely to get their values from the family.

What happens when a child becomes a teenager?

The teenage years can be an emotional assault course for all concerned. A gulf can grow between parents and their children during adolescence. One of the reasons many of us find it so hard is because it is a time of rapid physical development and deep emotional changes. These are exciting, but can also be confusing and uncomfortable for child and parent alike.

Parents often feel rejected, and in a sense they are. But this is often necessary for young people to develop their own identity. Even if you have rows and arguments, your children will usually think a lot of you. The rejections and conflicts are often not to do with your personality, but simply with the fact that you are parents, from whom your children must become independent if they are to have their own life.

As they become more independent, young people want to **try out new things**, but often recognise that they have little experience to fall back on when things get difficult. This may produce rapid changes in self-confidence and behaviour – feeling very adult one minute, very young and inexperienced the next.

> ✪ Being upset, feeling ill or lacking confidence can make your adolescent children feel vulnerable. They may show this with sulky behaviour rather than obvious distress. Parents have to be pretty flexible to deal with all this, and may feel under considerable strain themselves.

Adolescence is the time when people start in earnest to **learn about the world** and to find their place in it. This involves trying out new experiences, some of which may be risky or even dangerous. Young people can crave **excitement** in a way that most adults find difficult to understand – and exciting activities may be dangerous. Fortunately, most people manage to find their excitement in music, sport or other activities that involve a lot of energy but little real physical risk. When they do experiment – with drink or drugs or smoking – it is usually with friends. If a young person does this alone, they are in much greater danger. Warnings from older adolescents will usually be taken more seriously than those from parents.

What kind of difficulties can a young person have?

The young person can present with a number of difficulties, some of which are described below. If any of these seem to be severe or persistent, please refer to the relevant factsheets in this series.

It is important to note that despite the popular myth of 'difficult teenager', the majority of adolescents do not have significant or severe difficulties.

Emotional problems

- Overeating, excessive sleepiness and a persistent over-concern with appearance may be signs of **emotional distress**.
- **Anxiety** may produce phobias and panic attacks. Research suggests that emotional disorders are often not recognised, even by family and friends.
- At some time, four out of ten adolescents have felt so miserable that they have cried and have wanted to get away from everyone and everything. During their adolescence, more than one in five teenagers think so little of themselves that life does not seem worth living. In spite of these powerful feelings, **depression** may not be obvious to other people.

Sexual problems

The dramatic physical changes of adolescence can be very worrying to some teenagers, especially to those who are shy and who don't like to ask questions. At the other end of the scale, some express their concern with excessive bragging about sexual ability and experiences.

> ✪ Sensitive support, clear guidance and accurate information about different aspects of sex are essential, from parents, schools, GPs and family planning clinics.

- The age of consent for intercourse, both heterosexual and homosexual, is 16 in England, Scotland and Wales, and 17 in Northern Ireland. It is illegal to have sex if either partner is under this age, even if they give consent.
- More than half of young people in the UK will have had their first experience of sex before the age of 16, and so the risk of **pregnancy** is an important part of adolescent life. Research suggests that girls who are close to their parents are less likely to become pregnant in their teenage years.
- Those who start having sex early are at greater risk of early pregnancy and health problems. **Sexually transmitted diseases** are common, and HIV infection and AIDS are becoming ever more common.
- Most adolescents choose their partners quite carefully. Sleeping around and having risky, **unprotected intercourse** are often signs of underlying emotional problems. They may also be the signs of a risk-taking lifestyle – adolescents who take risks in one way tend to take risks in other ways as well.

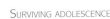

- Crushes on someone of the same gender are common in adolescence, but some young people are going to be **gay**. Some young people (and their parents) will not be sure whether they are gay or straight.
- Teenagers can get **confidential advice** on contraception from their GP who does not have to inform their parents. Emergency contraception from pharmacies is only available to those aged 16 or over.

Parental shock...

It can be surprisingly upsetting when your child has their first serious relationship, or you find out that they have started to have sex. For the first time in your life together, you are not the most important person to them. The sense of shock will pass, but you may need a while to adjust to the new state of affairs.

Behaviour problems

Teenagers and their parents complain about each other's behaviour. Parents often feel they have lost any sort of control or influence over their child. Adolescents want their parents to be clear and consistent about rules and boundaries, but at the same time may resent any restrictions on their growing freedom and ability to decide for themselves.

If disagreements are common and normal, when should you worry? Experience suggests that children are at a greater risk of getting into trouble if their parents don't know where they are. So, try to make sure that you know where they are going and what they are up to. If you really don't know, you need to find out.

School problems

If your child refuses to go to school, this can be because of:

- difficulties in separating from parents
- being a perfectionist, and becoming depressed because they can't do as well as they would want to
- disturbed family life, with early separation from or death of a parent
- an established pattern which may have started at primary school; these children often have physical symptoms, such as a headache or stomach ache.

> ✪ Bullying can cause problems at school. Around 1 in 10 secondary school children is bullied at some point; about 1 in 20 is bullied every week. If you are worried that this is happening, talk to the school to make sure that they enforce their anti-bullying policy.

Those who go to school, but then play truant, are usually unhappy at home and frustrated at school. They prefer to spend their days with others who feel the same way.

Emotional problems will often affect schoolwork – worrying about yourself or about what is going on at home makes it difficult to concentrate. Pressure to do well and to pass exams may come from parents or teachers, but adolescents usually want to do well and will push themselves. Excessive nagging can be counterproductive. Exams are important, but they should not be allowed to dominate life or to cause unhappiness.

Trouble with the law

- Most young people do not break the law. When they do, it usually only happens once.
- If a parent doesn't feel that breaking the law is particularly important, it is more likely that their children will offend.
- Unhappiness or distress can also lead to behaviour that will get adolescents into trouble with the police. It is always worth asking about their feelings if an adolescent is repeatedly getting into trouble.

Eating problems

Weight can be a real problem. If an adolescent is overweight and is criticised or made fun of, they are more likely to dislike themselves and to become depressed. This can lead to inactivity and comfort eating, which worsens the weight problem – dieting can actually aggravate the situation. It is more important to ensure that the young person feels happy with themselves, fat or thin.

Many adolescents diet. Fortunately, few will develop serious eating disorders – only around 1 in 100 teenagers develop anorexia, and 1 in 50 have bulimia. However, eating disorders are more likely to occur in those who take up serious dieting, think very little of themselves, are under stress and who have been overweight as children.

> ✪ Find out about any drugs your children may be using – see the telephone and web resources at the end of this toolkit.

Drugs, solvents and alcohol

- Many teenagers experiment with alcohol and illegal drugs. Around one in three 15-year-olds in England has used drugs at some time.

- Regular use of drugs or alcohol is much less common. Less than 1 in 100 of 11- to 12-year-olds regularly use drugs, but this increases to 1 in 6 of 15-year-olds.

- Although **cannabis** has been widely felt to be relatively harmless, there is now good evidence that it can make mental health problems worse in adolescence, and can double the risk of developing schizophrenia. Despite publicity about other drugs, **alcohol** is the most common drug to cause problems for adolescents.

- You should consider the possibility of drug or alcohol misuse when you notice sudden or dramatic changes in behaviour.

- **What if they ask about the drugs you used to use in your younger days?**

  Honesty is generally the best policy, although it is probably worth stressing the differences in drugs available now. For example, much of the cannabis available today is much stronger than what was available 20 years ago, and we now know a lot more about its risks to both physical and mental health.

Abuse

- Physical, emotional and sexual abuse may occur in adolescence and may cause many of the problems mentioned earlier. Children or teenagers who are being abused can find someone to talk to at ChildLine.

- Families with these problems need expert advice and should seek help. The list of organisations at the end of this toolkit may point you in the right direction.

Mental illness

Much less often, changes in behaviour and mood can mark the beginning of more serious psychiatric disorders. Although uncommon, **bipolar disorder** (manic depression) and **schizophrenia** may emerge for the first time during adolescence.

Extreme withdrawal may indicate schizophrenia, although there are usually other explanations for such behaviour. Parents who are concerned about these possibilities should ask to see their GP.

The good news for parents

Adolescence has had a bad press. However, recent studies have shown that most teenagers actually like their parents and feel that they get on well with them. Adolescence is a time when the process of growing up can help people to make positive changes, and to put the problems of the past behind them.

It is not just a difficult stage, although it can feel very much like it at times. The anxiety experienced by parents is more than matched by the periods of uncertainty, turmoil and unhappiness experienced by the adolescent.

> ✪ Most adolescents like their parents and get on well with them.

Difficult times come and go, but most adolescents don't develop serious problems. It is worth remembering this when things are difficult.

Parents may sometimes feel that they have failed. However, whatever may be said in the heat of the moment, they play a crucial part in their children's lives. Helping your children grow through adolescence can be profoundly satisfying.

Top tips

- **Don't be jealous**

  The good times and opportunities that adolescent children have may well make you feel very middle-aged. Their physical strength is increasing at a time that yours may well be waning. Jealousy can be the hidden fuel for all sorts of arguments and trouble.

- **Make your home a safe base**

  Adolescent children are exploring life, but need a base to come back to. Home should be somewhere they feel safe, where they will be protected, cared for and taken seriously.

- **Mutual support**

  Parents need to agree between themselves about their basic values and rules, and support each other in applying them. It is difficult for a teenager to respect parents who are always at each other's throats or undermining each other. A common trap is for one parent to ally themselves with their child against the other parent. This usually leads to constant trouble.

Easy listening

Adults need to be a source of **advice**, **sympathy** and **comfort**. A teenager needs to know that his or her parents will not automatically jump down their throat with a judgement, a criticism or routine advice. **Listening comes first.**

Rules

However fast they may be growing up, you are your children's providers and it is reasonable that you should decide what the ground rules are. Although adolescents may protest, **sensible rules** can be the basis for security and agreement. They must be:

- clear, so everybody knows where they stand
- where possible, they should be agreed with the children
- consistent, so everyone sticks to them
- reasonable
- less restrictive as children become more responsible.

You can't (and shouldn't) have rules for everything. Although some issues will not be negotiable, there should be room for bargaining on others.

> ✪ **Sanctions**, such as grounding or loss of pocket money, will only work if they are established in advance. Don't threaten these if you are not willing to carry them out. **Rewards** for behaving well are just as important – probably more important, in fact.

Managing disagreements

Involve your children in making family rules – like all of us, they are more likely to stick to rules if they can see some logic to them and have helped to make them. If a teenager is reluctant to discuss rules for him or herself, they may still do this if they can see that it might be helpful for younger brothers or sisters. If they don't want to get involved, they will just have to put up with the rules you decide on.

Parents should pick their battles. A lot of things adolescents do are irritating (as you probably irritate them too), but not all are worth an argument. It is usually better to spend time on praising good decisions or behaviour. Most annoying habits will burn themselves out once parents stop reacting to them.

Don't use corporal (physical) punishment

Although it is now viewed as unhelpful, many people still occasionally smack younger children. If you do this with adolescent children, you create the impression that violence is an acceptable way to solve difficulties. This means that they are more likely to grow up to use violence as adults. You can get stuck in a cycle of violence – you hit them, they hit you back (because they are now big enough), you hit them again and so on.

Set the example

Although they are becoming more independent, your children will still learn a lot about how to behave from you. If you don't want them to swear, don't swear yourself. If you don't want them to get drunk, don't get drunk yourself. If you don't want them to be violent, don't use violence yourself. If you want them to be kind and generous to other people, try to be like this yourself. 'Do as I say, not as I do' just won't work.

Gratitude

Don't worry if your children aren't as grateful as you would like. It's great if they are, but they may not be until they have children of their own and realise how demanding it can be.

When all else fails, get help

Sometimes, all of this may not be enough and you (or your child) may be unable to cope. Worries about the physical changes of adolescence – are they too early, too late or ever going to happen – or about relationships can be discussed with your **GP**.

> ✪ If there is violence in your family – parents hitting one another, children hitting each other, parents hitting children or children hitting parents – ask for help.

When problems arise at school, obviously **teachers** may be a useful source of information. The teacher may suggest that an educational psychologist becomes involved. Psychologists can find out if there are any particular problems with learning, but can also offer counselling if relationships are the issue.

Adolescents who experience turmoil or distress for more than a few months – persistent depression, anxiety, serious eating disorders or difficult behaviour – generally require outside help. **Counselling** agencies may be suitable if things have not gone too far. They exist for young people and for parents and some contact addresses are listed overleaf. However, specialist help may be needed from the child and adolescent mental health services (**CAMHS**). They mainly offer out-patient treatment and can be contacted through your GP.

As they grow older, your children will want more privacy. Adolescents may, quite naturally, wish to see the doctor on their own. The law allows them to agree their own treatment from the age of 16, or younger under certain circumstances.

Recommended reading

Other factsheets in this series:
Good parenting, Drugs and alcohol, Domestic violence, Behavioural problems and conduct disorder, CAMHS

The Young Mind: An Essential Guide to Mental Health for Young Adults, Parents and Teachers, edited by Sue Bailey and Mike Shooter (2009) – an accessible, user-friendly handbook produced by the Royal College of Psychiatrists.

References

Gutman LM, Brown J, Akerman R, et al. *Change in Wellbeing from Childhood to Adolescence: Risk and Resilience*. Centre for Research on the Wider Benefits of Learning, Institute of Education, 2010.

Rutter M, Bishop D, Pine D, et al (eds) *Rutter's Child and Adolescent Psychiatry* (5th edn). Wiley–Blackwell, 2008.

Useful websites

- **Brook**: www.brook.org.uk; provides a free and confidential sexual, health and contraception advice by young people up to the age of 25. Helpline: 0808 802 1234.

- **ChildLine**: www.childline.org.uk; a free and confidential service for children. Helpline 0800 1111.

- **Kidscape**: www.kidscape.org.uk; advice, training courses and helpful booklets and information about bullying.

- **Family Lives**: http://familylives.org.uk; help and advice to parents bringing up children and teenagers. Helpline: 0808 800 2222.

- **Talk to Frank**: www.talktofrank.com; free and confidential drugs information and advice line. Helpline: 0800 776600.

- **Young Minds**: www.youngminds.org.uk; free advice and support for parents worried about their children's behaviour, emotional problems and mental health. Parents' helpline: 0808 802 5544.

- **Your Teenager**: www.yourteenager.co.uk; website which focuses on how to handle teenage behaviour and build a positive parent/teen relationship.

- **Directgov**: www.direct.gov.uk; lots of useful information on public services and also gives information on some common parental concerns.

Notes

_____

_____

_____

_____

_____

_____

_____

_____